2021
国际医学教育研究前沿报告

International Medical Education Research Fronts Report

闻德亮　李鸿鹤　著

科学出版社
北　京

内 容 简 介

医学教育国际化的不断发展，要求越来越多的医学院校和专家学者加强对医学教育发展的认识，及时更新国际先进教育教学理念。本报告通过文献计量学和文本挖掘的最新技术，基于 Web of Science 数据库，全面梳理了 2020 年度的全球医学教育发展状态，追踪全球医学教育研究领域的最新发展变化；按照临床医生岗位胜任力分类，探讨医学知识与终身学习、临床技能与医疗服务、疾病预防与健康促进、信息与管理、人际沟通、团队合作、科学研究、核心价值观与职业素养八大要素的热点前沿；聚焦全球医学教育技术，分析医学教育技术版块的发展特征和热点趋势；构建医学教育领域专有的 ESI 统计排名；解析国际医学教育研究期刊。在本年度的研究前沿报告中，与时俱进地增设了关于国际上重点新兴议题"新冠肺炎疫情下的医学教育变革"专题介绍。通过这样的平台与数据信息，以期能够帮助全球的医学教育研究者、工作者紧跟时代步伐，共促医学教育的长足发展。

图书在版编目（CIP）数据

2021 国际医学教育研究前沿报告 / 闻德亮，李鸿鹤著 . —北京：科学出版社，2021.9

ISBN 978-7-03-069750-9

Ⅰ . ① 2… Ⅱ . ①闻… ②李… Ⅲ . ①医学教育 – 研究报告 – 世界 – 2021 Ⅳ . ① R-4

中国版本图书馆 CIP 数据核字（2021）第 187500 号

责任编辑：王　颖 / 责任校对：宁辉彩
责任印制：李　彤 / 封面设计：陈　敬

科学出版社 出版
北京东黄城根北街 16 号
邮政编码：100717
http: // www.sciencep.com

北京建宏印刷有限公司 印刷
科学出版社发行　各地新华书店经销

*

2021 年 9 月第　一　版　开本：720 × 1000　1/16
2022 年 1 月第二次印刷　印张：5 1/4
字数：100 000

定价：**45.00 元**
（如有印装质量问题，我社负责调换）

序

  建设教育强国是中华民族伟大复兴的基础工程；人民健康是民族昌盛和国家富强的重要标志。因此，培养高水平医学人才是全球高等医学教育机构的时代担当。随着全球化发展不断深入，全球医学教育事业和卫生健康事业都进入了一个新的历史发展阶段。如何在相互依存的世界里实现更好的医学教育，要求全球的医学教育研究者、工作者紧跟医学教育脉搏，加强互相了解，及时更新教育教学理念，与世界发展共频。

  中国医科大学作为中国较早开展西医学学院式教育的高等学校，始终致力于为人类卫生健康事业发展做出积极贡献，在高等医学教育研究与改革方面积累了丰富的经验。中国医科大学国际医学教育研究院经过30余年的探索与发展，借鉴国际先进医学教育理念和经验，结合中国国情进行研究实践，取得了具有中国特色的医学教育改革和研究成果，并将成果推广应用。作为以"育人为本，国际视野，立足国情，服务社会"为使命的国际化医学教育研究机构，有责任也有义务向国家宏观决策层、专家学者和社会全面系统地报告国际医学教育研究的发展情况，对未来发展进行前瞻性的思考和展望。

  为更好地融入并推动医学教育的理论研究和改革发展，我们迫切需要一部全球医学教育发展指南来指导中国的医学教育工作者从事医疗教育实践的教学与研究，《国际医学教育研究前沿报告》正是利用这一契机编写的一部具有前沿意义的医学教育发展指南，为国内外众多医学院校和专家学者提供了追踪全球医学教育整体态势和发展变化的机会。

  本研究报告的发布离不开科睿唯安团队的通力合作与科学出版社的大力支持。我们在编写过程中力争保证资料的全面性和准确性。参与该项目的专家学者们召开了一系列的研讨会、审稿会等，将撰写的每一个细节力争做到最好。但也由于精力和编写能力有限，本研究报告中的问题和失当之处在所难免，恳切希望各位同道和读者批评指正。

闻德亮

2020 年 4 月 2 日

前　言

医学教育是卫生健康事业发展的重要基石。党的十八大以来，我国医学教育蓬勃发展，为卫生健康事业输送了大批高素质医学人才。2021年正值"十四五"开局之年，面对新冠疫情提出的新挑战、实施健康中国战略的新任务、世界医学发展的新要求，迫切需要一部关于国内外医学教育的发展指南来帮助我国的医学教育工作者更好地从事医学教育实践的教学和研究，推进医学教育创新发展。《国际医学教育研究前沿报告》历年版本系列书的出版恰逢其时，是一部具有先进指导意义的医学教育发展指南。本系列书对医学教育领域整体态势及发展变化做出了综合概括描述，利用科学计量学技术揭示国际上医学教育研究的发展特征和研究热点，进而把握国际医学教育的动态发展变化。

《国际医学教育研究前沿报告》历年版本系列书自2018年至今已走过四个春秋，内容不断地更新和丰富，同时也更加关注医学人才的培养要求和质量。今年，我们在延续原有内容版块和主导思想的基础上，针对新冠疫情影响下的医学教育变革、医学人才培养要求和广大读者的期待，在书中新增添了三部分内容，多角度探索医学教育研究的发展脉络。这三部分分别是全球医学教育技术研究专题分析，临床医生岗位胜任力前沿分析，以及国际上重点新兴议题"新冠肺炎疫情下的医学教育变革"的专题介绍。

至此，《2021国际医学教育研究前沿报告》已经涵盖了医学教育研究论文外部特征描绘、热点研究主题内容挖掘和聚类分析、临床医生岗位胜任力八大要素的前沿分析、国际新兴议题和热点专题介绍、国际医学教育研究机构ESI排名和国际期刊统计分析等全面丰富的内容版块，旨在为国内外医学教育工作者提供完整的研究概况，助力以胜任力为导向的全球第三代医学教育改革，特别是为全球医学教育技术工作者和受新冠疫情影响的医学教育工作者提供明确的研究热点和前沿方向。本书通过揭示全球医学教育的研究现状和热点前沿，从而帮助全球的医学教育工作者紧跟国际医学教育整体发展态势，并对未来发展进行前瞻性的思考和展望，使得处于疫情防控常态化形势下的医学教育变得有迹可循、有理可依。

最后要感谢中国医科大学编者团队——曲波教授、崔雷教授、赵阳助理研究员，以及国际医学教育研究院的博、硕士研究生宋鑫智、江南、崔雪梅、辛春雨等的辛勤工作，以及科睿唯安团队的大力支持，我们坚信《国际医学教育研究前沿报告》历年版本系列书将对全球医学教育的改革发展大有裨益，在未来的发展中一定会越办越好！

闻德亮

2021年6月17日

目　　录

2021 国际医学教育研究前沿报告

（中文部分）

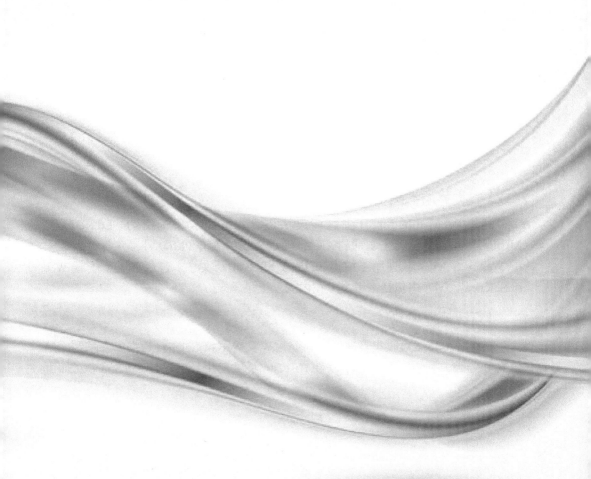

背　景

医学教育的国际化进程逐步加快，形成了全球性的相互依存，这种趋势要求我们必须加强互相了解，及时更新理念，掌握国际医学教育研究的现状和发展趋势，从而不断开拓医学教育研究与改革的新未来。2018—2020 年我们连续三年发布了国际医学教育研究系列前沿报告，在国内外医学教育界引起了强烈反响。2021 年，我们在延续去年原有内容版块的基础上，对临床医生岗位胜任力研究前沿进行了系统解析，并进行了关于全球医学教育技术的专题探讨。我们希望通过这样一个平台，能够帮助全球的医学教育研究者、工作者紧跟时代步伐，把握国际医学教育的整体发展态势，对未来发展进行前瞻性的思考和展望。

目　的

（1）基于 Web of Science 数据库，全面梳理 2019—2020 年度全球医学教育发展状态。

（2）探讨临床医生岗位胜任力八大要素的热点前沿。

（3）聚焦全球医学教育技术，分析医学教育技术研究版块的热点和发展趋势。

（4）构建医学教育研究领域 ESI 机构统计排名。

（5）描绘医学教育研究期刊外部特征和发表兴趣取向，为医学教育研究者提供参考。

方　法

（一）数据采集

利用 PubMed 的 MeSH 主题词方法进行检索，收集标引为 "Education, Medical" 及其下位类主题词的文献，确定文献的独有 PMID 号，并与科睿唯安的 Web of Science 数据库（均为 SCIE 或 SSCI 收录文章）进行匹配，下载 Web of Science 数据库中包括参考文献在内的全记录题录。

（二）文献概览

在第一步数据集收集整理的基础上，基于 Web of Science 数据库文献题录的信息和分类，利用科学计量学软件 HistCite 及可视化分析工具 CiteSpace 对如下指标进行统计分析,包括:高发文量国家(地区)分布、高被引量国家(地区)分布、高发文量机构分布、高被引量机构分布、高发文量作者分布、高被引量作者分布、高发文量期刊分布和高被引量期刊分布。

(三)研究前沿

1. 高频主题词分布及聚类分析

在上述数据集收集整理的基础上,利用书目共现分析系统 BICOMB 对来源文献的 MeSH Terms 字段进行主要主题词提取,生成高频主题词列表。高频主题词聚类通过将生成的高频主题词词篇矩阵导入聚类工具 gCLUTO 实现。

2. 引文共被引聚类分析

引文共被引聚类是通过对共同出现在施引文献中的被引文献间关系的分析来反映被引文献间聚集程度的一种聚类方式。本研究基于书目共现分析系统 Bicomb 对纳入本次分析的文献集的引文进行抽取、排序并生成共被引矩阵,最终进行聚类分析。

结　　果

一、国际医学教育研究文献概览及研究前沿分析

检索策略:MeSH 主题词"Education,Medical"+ JCR 数据库中教育门类下 10 种医学教育期刊(*Academic Medicine* / *Medical Education* / *Medical Teacher* / *BMC Medical Education* / *Journal of Surgical Education* / *Advances in Health Sciences Education* / *Teaching and Learning in Medicine* / *Medical Education Online* / *Anatomical Sciences Education* / *Academic Psychiatry*)。

检索时间范围:因为数据库收录文献存在延迟现象,所以往往当年的文献统计量并未代表该年度发表论文的最终数量,需要再合并入上一年度的发文数量进行补充,施行轮动制的年限覆盖范围的分析。因此,第一部分国际医学教育研究文献概览纳入了 2019—2020 年度两年的文献用于分析目前全球医学教育的发展状态(注:在《2020 国际医学教育研究前沿报告》中,2019 年的文献数据因为文献收录延迟问题,也并未纳入完全,因此通过这样的方法,实现对上一年度遗漏文献的补充)。

1. 国际医学教育论文 2019—2020 年发文量及被引量的国家 / 地区分布（图 1）

序号	国家 / 地区	发文量	百分比	序号	国家 / 地区	被引量	百分比	平均被引量
1	USA	6531	54.88	1	USA	14726	40.12	2.25
2	UK	1352	11.36	2	UK	3133	8.54	2.32
3	Canada	1141	9.59	3	Canada	3043	8.29	2.67
4	Australia	639	5.37	4	Netherlands	1836	5	3.57
5	Netherlands	514	4.32	5	Australia	1759	4.79	2.75
6	Germany	451	3.79	6	Germany	1192	3.25	2.64
7	PRC	359	3.02	7	Italy	827	2.25	4.07
8	France	217	1.82	8	PRC	746	2.03	2.08
9	Italy	203	1.71	9	France	595	1.62	2.74
10	Switzerland	167	1.40	10	Singapore	556	1.51	4.09
11	India	164	1.38	11	Spain	460	1.25	3.13
12	Brazil	162	1.36	12	Sweden	444	1.21	4.58
13	Spain	147	1.24	13	Belgium	426	1.16	4.95
14	Singapore	136	1.14	14	Ireland	409	1.11	3.53
15	Japan	128	1.08	15	New Zealand	389	1.06	3.60

图 1　国际医学教育论文 2019—2020 年发文量及被引量的国家 / 地区分布

2. 国际医学教育论文 2019—2020 年发文量及被引量的机构分布（图 2）

序号	机构	发文量	百分比	序号	机构	被引量	百分比	平均被引量
1	Harvard Med Sch	455	3.82	1	Harvard Med Sch	1320	1.51	2.90
2	Univ of Toronto	342	2.87	2	Univ of Calif San Francisco	1209	1.39	3.61
3	Univ of Calif San Francisco	335	2.82	3	Univ of Michigan	948	1.09	3.11
4	Univ of Michigan	305	2.56	4	Univ of Penn	946	1.09	4.28
5	Mayo Clin	261	2.19	5	Univ of Toronto	928	1.06	2.71
6	Stanford Univ	261	2.19	6	Mayo Clin	911	1.05	3.49
7	Univ of Penn	221	1.86	7	Univ of Washington	824	0.95	3.75
8	Univ of Washington	220	1.85	8	Northwestern Univ	807	0.93	4.41
9	Johns Hopkins Univ	203	1.71	9	Stanford Univ	793	0.91	3.04
10	Maastricht Univ	190	1.60	10	Uniformed Serv Univ of Hlth Sci	609	0.7	4.17
11	Massachusetts Gen Hosp	187	1.57	11	Maastricht Univ	607	0.7	3.19
12	Northwestern Univ	183	1.54	12	Johns Hopkins Univ	587	0.67	2.89
13	Univ of British Columbia	165	1.39	13	Duke Univ	522	0.6	3.46
14	Brigham & Women's Hosp	152	1.28	14	Univ of British Columbia	512	0.59	3.10
15	Duke Univ	151	1.27	15	Massachusetts Gen Hosp	475	0.55	2.54

图 2　国际医学教育论文 2019—2020 年发文量及被引量的机构分布

3. 国际医学教育论文 2019—2020 年发文量及被引量的作者分布（图 3）

序号	高发文作者	所在机构	发文量	序号	高被引作者	所在机构	被引量	平均被引量
1	Durning, Steven J.	Uniformed Serv Univ of Hlth Sci	46	1	Rose, Suzanne	Univ of Penn	198	39.60
2	Sally A. Santen	Virginia Commonwealth Univ	38	2	Durning, Steven J.	Uniformed Serv Univ of Hlth Sci	176	3.83
3	Ten Cate, Olle	Univ Med Ctr Utrecht	34	3	Ten Cate, Olle	Univ of Med Ctr Utrecht	168	4.94
4	Park, Yoon Soo	Univ of Illinois	31	4	Bilimoria, Karl Y.	Northwestern Univ	157	9.24
5	Cleland, Jennifer	Univ of Aberdeen	29	5	Esperto, Francesco	Campus Biomed Univ	151	18.88
6	Varpio, Lara	Uniformed Serv Univ of Hlth Sci	26	6	Ginsburg, Shiphra	Univ of Toronto	146	8.11
7	Hauer, Karen E.	Univ of Calif San Francisco	23	7	Yue-Yung Hu	Northwestern Univ	141	11.75
8	Roberts, Laura Weiss	Stanford Univ	23	8	Buyske, Jo	Amer Board Surg	135	19.29
9	Sandhu, Gurjit	Univ of Michigan Hlth Syst	21	9	Hoyt, David B.	Amer Coll Surg	135	22.50
10	Balon, Richard	Wayne State Univ	19	10	Ellis, Ryan J.	Northwestern Univ	130	16.25
11	Dornan, Tim	Queens Univ Belfast	19	11	Hewitt, D. Brock	Northwestern Univ	128	21.33
12	Eva, Kevin W.	Univ of British Columbia	19	12	Duma, Narjust	Mayo Clin	127	63.50
13	Konge, Lars	Univ Copenhagen	19	13	Varpio, Lara	Uniformed Serv Univ of Hlth Sci	126	4.85
14	Teunissen, Pim W.	Maastricht Univ	19	14	Molina, Julian R.	Mayo Clin	126	126.00
15	Ginsburg, Shiphra	Univ of Toronto	18	15	Santana-Davila	Univ of Washington	126	126.00

图 3 国际医学教育论文 2019—2020 年发文量及被引量的作者分布

注：作者分布统计对所有发文作者的贡献同等对待，不区分第一作者、通信作者与合著作者

4. 国际医学教育论文 2019—2020 年高频主题词分布（图 4）

序号	主题词	频次	百分比	序号	主题词	频次	百分比
1	Internship and Residency	3986	7.60	21	Pediatrics	355	0.68
2	Students, Medical	2112	4.03	22	Teaching	348	0.66
3	Education, Medical	1983	3.78	23	Psychiatry	347	0.66
4	Education, Medical, Graduate	1650	3.15	24	Surgeons	334	0.64
5	Clinical Competence	1601	3.05	25	Career Choice	331	0.63
6	Education, Medical, Undergraduate	1453	2.77	26	Fellowships and Scholarships	289	0.55
7	Curriculum	1056	2.01	27	Emergency Medicine	277	0.53
8	Physicians	624	1.19	28	Education, Distance	276	0.53
9	Coronavirus Infections	615	1.17	29	Burnout, Professional	272	0.52
10	Pneumonia, Viral	612	1.17	30	Radiology	272	0.52
11	General Surgery	601	1.15	31	Clinical Clerkship	269	0.51
12	Educational Measurement	581	1.11	32	Internal Medicine	250	0.48
13	Simulation Training	502	0.96	33	Anatomy	239	0.46
14	Education, Medical, Continuing	443	0.84	34	Problem-Based Learning	236	0.45
15	Faculty, Medical	426	0.81	35	Physician-Patient Relations	220	0.42
16	Pandemics	426	0.81	36	Biomedical Research	215	0.41
17	Attitude of Health Personnel	417	0.80	37	Betacoronavirus	215	0.41
18	COVID-19	381	0.73	38	Communication	212	0.40
19	Schools, Medical	375	0.72	39	Orthopedics	210	0.40
20	Learning	370	0.71	40	Health Personnel	206	0.39

图 4 国际医学教育论文 2019—2020 年高频主题词分布

5. 国际医学教育论文 2019—2020 年高频主题词聚类（图 5）

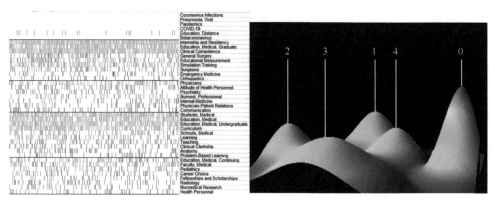

图 5　国际医学教育论文 2019—2020 年高频主题词聚类

注：右图中数字表示高频主题词聚类所形成的主题类别

通过高频主题词聚类分析，2019—2020 年国际医学教育研究主题涵盖以下 5 个主要方面：

（1）新冠肺炎疫情影响下远程教学在医学教育教学中的作用。

（2）标准化病人和虚拟仿真在住院医师规范化培训中的应用。

（3）医务人员临床沟通技能的培养与评价。

（4）人体解剖学课程教与学模式的改革。

（5）其他，包括医务工作者的职业选择，绩效分配等。

新兴专题：新冠肺炎疫情下的医学教育变革

检索策略：MeSH 主题词"Education，Medical"＋JCR 数据库中教育门类下 10 种医学教育期刊（*Academic Medicine / Medical Education / Medical Teacher / BMC Medical Education / Journal of Surgical Education / Advances in Health Sciences Education / Teaching and Learning in Medicine / Medical Education Online / Anatomical Sciences Education / Academic Psychiatry*）AND MeSH 主题词"COVID-19"。

1. 新冠肺炎疫情下国际医学教育论文 2019—2020 年高频主题词分布（图 6 ）

序号	主题词	频次	百分比	序号	主题词	频次	百分比
1	Coronavirus Infections	599	8.81	21	Educational Measurement	37	0.54
2	Pneumonia, Viral	596	8.77	22	Dermatology	36	0.53
3	COVID-19	584	8.59	23	Radiology	36	0.53
4	Pandemics	465	6.84	24	Schools, Medical	34	0.50
5	Internship and Residency	422	6.21	25	Ophthalmology	34	0.50
6	Education, Medical	290	4.27	26	Urology	33	0.49
7	Education, Distance	235	3.46	27	Delivery of Health Care	31	0.46
8	Betacoronavirus	211	3.10	28	Anatomy	31	0.46
9	Education, Medical, Graduate	204	3.00	29	Otolaryngology	31	0.46
10	Students, Medical	202	2.97	30	Teaching	30	0.44
11	Education, Medical, Undergraduate	139	2.04	31	Neurosurgery	30	0.44
12	Telemedicine	78	1.15	32	Infection Control	30	0.44
13	Curriculum	68	1.00	33	Physicians	30	0.44
14	Clinical Competence	67	0.99	34	Clinical Clerkship	27	0.40
15	General Surgery	63	0.93	35	Personnel Selection	27	0.40
16	SARS-CoV-2	57	0.84	36	Faculty, Medical	25	0.37
17	Computer-Assisted Instruction	48	0.71	37	Pediatrics	25	0.37
18	Videoconferencing	42	0.62	38	Interviews as Topic	24	0.35
19	Education, Medical, Continuing	39	0.57	39	Surgery, Plastic	22	0.32
20	Fellowships and Scholarships	38	0.56	40	Simulation Training	22	0.32

图 6　新冠肺炎疫情下国际医学教育论文 2019—2020 年高频主题词分布

2. 新冠肺炎疫情下国际医学教育论文 2019—2020 年前 1% 高频被引论文（图 7）

序号	高频被引论文	被引频次
1	Rose S. Medical Student Education in the Time of COVID-19. JAMA. 2020 Jun 2;323(21):2131-2132.	200
2	Chick R C, Clifton G T, Peace K M, Propper B W, Hale D F, Alseidi A A, Vreeland T J. Using Technology to Maintain the Education of Residents During the COVID-19 Pandemic. J Surg Educ. 2020 Jul-Aug;77(4):729-732.	117
3	Fix O K, Hameed B, Fontana R J, Kwok R M, McGuire B M, Mulligan D C, Pratt D S, Russo M W, Schilsky M L, Verna E C, Loomba R, Cohen D E, Bezerra J A, Reddy K R, Chung R T. Clinical Best Practice Advice for Hepatology and Liver Transplant Providers During the COVID-19 Pandemic: AASLD Expert Panel Consensus Statement. Hepatology. 2020 Jul;72(1):287-304.	89
4	Ahmed H, Allaf M, Elghazaly H. COVID-19 and medical education. Lancet Infect Dis. 2020 Jul;20(7):777-778.	80
5	Almarzooq Z I, Lopes M, Kochar A. Virtual Learning During the COVID-19 Pandemic: A Disruptive Technology in Graduate Medical Education. J Am Coll Cardiol. 2020 May 26;75(20):2635-2638.	60
6	Porpiglia F, Checcucci E, Amparore D, Verri P, Campi R, Claps F, Esperto F, Fiori C, Carrieri G, Ficarra V, Mario Scarpa R, Dasgupta P. Slowdown of urology residents' learning curve during the COVID-19 emergency. BJU Int. 2020 Jun;125(6):e15-e17.	52
7	Amparore D, Claps F, Cacciamani G E, Esperto F, Fiori C, Liguori G, Serni S, Trombetta C, Carini M, Porpiglia F, Checcucci E, Campi R. Impact of the COVID-19 pandemic on urology residency training in Italy. Minerva Urol Nefrol. 2020 Aug;72(4):505-509.	52
8	Kogan M, Klein S E, Hannon C P, Nolte M T. Orthopaedic Education During the COVID-19 Pandemic. J Am Acad Orthop Surg. 2020 Jun 1;28(11):e456-e464.	50
9	Evans D J R, Bay B H, Wilson T D, Smith C F, Lachman N, Pawlina W. Going Virtual to Support Anatomy Education: A STOPGAP in the Midst of the Covid-19 Pandemic. Anat Sci Educ. 2020 May;13(3):279-283.	49
10	Nassar A H, Zern N K, McIntyre L K, Lynge D, Smith C A, Petersen R P, Horvath K D, Wood D E. Emergency Restructuring of a General Surgery Residency Program During the Coronavirus Disease 2019 Pandemic: The University of Washington Experience. JAMA Surg. 2020 Jul 1;155(7):624-627.	48
11	Alvin M D, George E, Deng F, Warhadpande S, Lee SI. The Impact of COVID-19 on Radiology Trainees. Radiology. 2020 Aug;296(2):246-248.	48
12	Pather N, Blyth P, Chapman J A, Dayal M R, Flack N A M S, Fogg Q A, Green R A, Hulme A K, Johnson I P, Meyer A J, Morley J W, Shortland P J, Štrkalj G, Štrkalj M, Valter K, Webb A L, Woodley S J, Lazarus M D. Forced Disruption of Anatomy Education in Australia and New Zealand: An Acute Response to the Covid-19 Pandemic. Anat Sci Educ. 2020 May;13(3):284-300.	47
13	Dedeilia A, Sotiropoulos M G, Hanrahan J G, Janga D, Dedeilias P, Sideris M. Medical and Surgical Education Challenges and Innovations in the COVID-19 Era: A Systematic Review. In Vivo. 2020 Jun;34(3 Suppl):1603-1611.	45
14	Ripp J, Peccoralo L, Charney D. Attending to the Emotional Well-Being of the Health Care Workforce in a New York City Health System During the COVID-19 Pandemic. Acad Med. 2020 Aug;95(8):1136-1139.	41

图 7　新冠肺炎疫情下国际医学教育论文 2019—2020 年前 1% 高频被引论文

3. 新冠肺炎疫情下国际医学教育论文 2019—2020 年高频主题词聚类（图 8）

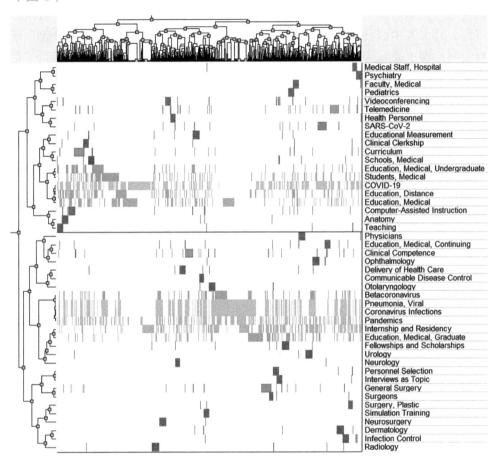

图 8　新冠肺炎疫情下国际医学教育论文 2019—2020 年高频主题词聚类

通过高频主题词聚类分析，2019—2020 年新冠肺炎疫情下国际医学教育研究主题涵盖以下 2 个主要方面：

（1）新冠肺炎疫情对本科医学教育（医学院校教育）的影响。

（2）新冠肺炎疫情对临床实践（毕业后医学教育和继续医学教育）的影响。

新冠肺炎疫情下的医学教育挑战分析

新冠肺炎疫情是对我国医学教育供给水平和支撑能力的一次"大考""严考"，揭示出当前我国医学教育面临的诸多挑战，但从"危"与"机"并存的辩证角度来看，不失为一个倒逼医学教育改革发展的有利契机。

（1）医师资源始终存在非均衡性分布状态

新冠肺炎疫情凸显了我国医师资源的不协调特征，各省区市之间和城乡之间的发展水平差异明显，拔尖创新医学人才供给匮乏。第一，医师供需匹配存在区域性差别问题。北京、浙江和上海等东部地区医师数量相对充足，云南、广西、甘肃等中西部地区的数量相对短缺。第二，医师群体的"两极分化"现象明显。即中心城市和三级医院相对集中，广大城乡基层地区的医师数量"捉襟见肘"，农村每千人口医师数仅为城市每千人口医师数的45%。第三，受传统的计划性招生制度影响，临床医学专业的高层次拔尖创新人才培养能力欠缺。我国临床医学八年制本博连读专业的招生规模较小，具备招生资格的大学不多。目前仅有14所大学可以招收八年制学生，且各校每年八年制实际招收人数占医学招生比例较低。

（2）医疗卫生事业的发展环境存在"隐患"

新冠肺炎疫情折射出政府财政投入不高、医生受尊重不够等掣肘医疗卫生发展的环境问题。第一，医疗卫生领域的财政投入仍需增加。相较于美国、日本等发达国家，我国医疗卫生支出占政府总支出比重较小，卫生总费用占GDP的比重较小且处于相对落后状况。第二，大学人才培养的政府投入不足，且部属高校和地方高校之间的经费差距较大。第三，医生的社会地位和尊医重医的社会风气亟待提升和形成。医患关系的平等性丧失和医生社会地位的逐渐下降，极大地削弱了医学教育尤其是临床医生的吸引力、培养力和输送力。

（3）公共卫生体系的规划建设缺乏足够重视

新冠肺炎疫情暴露了我国公共卫生管理体制机制的难点，疾病预防控制机构的规模不大、力量不足等支持力问题，尤其是从业人员专业性不强和人才流失压力更成为制约公共卫生体系防疫抗疫作用发挥的主要瓶颈。第一，公共卫生事业的管理体制机制束缚，一定程度地挤压和削弱了专业机构的发展空间及关键话语权。第二，我国疾病预防控制机构数量与从业人员储备均呈现"不增反降"的趋势，致使疫情期间出现大量"突击"招人的现象。第三，公共卫生医师流失现象堪忧。薪资收入偏低、职业归属感遗失已成为高学历毕业生和公共卫生执业医师"不愿来""留不住""不好留"的主要原因。

（4）医学人才的培养过程存在薄弱环节

新冠肺炎疫情中令人痛心疾首的医护感染揭示了面向"大健康""全周期"医学培养系统的不充分和不全面，临床医学人才的公共卫生基础知识和新发传染病防控技能等方面漏洞亟待弥补。第一，临床医学人才培养过程中普遍存在的重"治疗"轻"预防"知识结构失调，以及重"技术"轻"防护"的实践能力短板。第二，公共卫生与预防医学人才的专业培养存在明显的"医防脱节"现象，尤其是防疫抗病的实践能力始终薄弱。

未来时期，全面提升临床医生的多样化供给能力，多举措提高医学教育供给质量，重构公共卫生体系的安全防护力与公信力，优化医学教育的外部治理机制，成为深化医学教育改革、加快医学教育创新发展的主要路径。

本专题介绍部分取自：闻德亮．由新冠肺炎疫情防控引发的医学教育思考 [J]. 中国高教研究，2020(5): 43-47, 77.

二、临床医生岗位胜任力前沿分析

（一）医学知识与终身学习

检索策略：（Knowledge [MeSH] OR Learning [MeSH]）AND（Physicians [MeSH] OR Internship and Residency [MeSH] OR Students，Medical [MeSH]）。
统计年限：2011 年 1 月 1 日至 2020 年 12 月 31 日。

1. 医学知识与终身学习 2011—2020 年高频主题词分布（图 9）

序号	主题词	频次	百分比	序号	主题词	频次	百分比
1	Students, Medical	2206	8.80	21	Computer-Assisted Instruction	179	0.71
2	Learning	1219	4.86	22	Clinical Clerkship	176	0.70
3	Internship and Residency	1155	4.61	23	Formative Feedback	176	0.70
4	Education, Medical, Undergraduate	1148	4.58	24	Schools, Medical	137	0.55
5	Clinical Competence	1064	4.24	25	Education, Medical, Continuing	134	0.53
6	Problem-Based Learning	772	3.08	26	Communication	128	0.51
7	Education, Medical	602	2.40	27	Physician-Patient Relations	128	0.51
8	Teaching	566	2.26	28	Pediatrics	128	0.51
9	Education, Medical, Graduate	481	1.92	29	Interprofessional Relations	126	0.50
10	Educational Measurement	432	1.72	30	Computer Simulation	112	0.45
11	Curriculum	430	1.71	31	General Practitioners	110	0.44
12	Physicians	423	1.69	32	Peer Group	106	0.42
13	Learning Curve	295	1.18	33	Knowledge	99	0.39
14	Surgeons	247	0.98	34	Internal Medicine	98	0.39
15	Attitude of Health Personnel	236	0.94	35	Problem Solving	94	0.37
16	General Surgery	211	0.84	36	Emergency Medicine	92	0.37
17	Anatomy	198	0.79	37	Internet	90	0.36
18	Faculty, Medical	196	0.78	38	Health Knowledge, Attitudes, Practice	89	0.35
19	Laparoscopy	189	0.75	39	Robotic Surgical Procedures	89	0.35
20	Simulation Training	184	0.73	40	Anesthesiology	87	0.35

图 9　医学知识与终身学习 2011—2020 年高频主题词分布

2. 医学知识与终身学习 2011—2020 年高频主题词聚类（图 10）

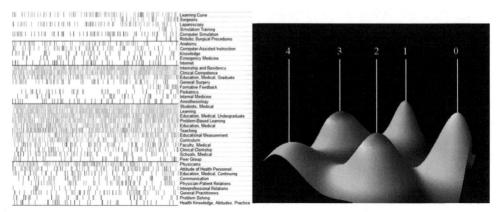

图 10　医学知识与终身学习 2011—2020 年高频主题词聚类

注：右图中数字表示高频主题词聚类所形成的主题类别

通过高频主题词聚类分析，近 10 年医学知识与终身学习研究主题涵盖以下 5 个主要方面：

（1）机器人辅助手术对外科医师学习曲线的影响。

（2）网络教学资源在人体解剖学课程教学中的应用。

（3）关于住培医师临床技能培训效果的研究。

（4）PBL、同伴互助学习等教学方法在医学教育中的应用及效果评价研究。

（5）其他，包括跨专业教育、职业困境解决方案等。

（二）临床技能与医疗服务

检索策略：（Clinical Competence [Majr：NoExp] OR Patient Care [Majr：NoExp]）AND（Physicians [MeSH] OR Internship and Residency [MeSH] OR Students，Medical [MeSH]）。

统计年限：2011 年 1 月 1 日至 2020 年 12 月 31 日。

1. 临床技能与医疗服务 2011—2020 年高频主题词分布（图 11）

序号	主题词	频次	百分比	序号	主题词	频次	百分比
1	Clinical Competence	8501	19.32	21	General Practitioners	236	0.54
2	Internship and Residency	3202	7.28	22	Education, Medical, Continuing	226	0.51
3	Students, Medical	1412	3.21	23	Communication	222	0.50
4	Physicians	1233	2.80	24	Physician-Patient Relations	215	0.49
5	Education, Medical, Graduate	1187	2.70	25	Teaching	206	0.47
6	Educational Measurement	878	2.00	26	Clinical Clerkship	203	0.46
7	Education, Medical, Undergraduate	719	1.63	27	Anesthesiology	194	0.44
8	General Surgery	645	1.47	28	Competency-Based Education	193	0.44
9	Curriculum	542	1.23	29	Practice Patterns, Physicians'	184	0.42
10	Attitude of Health Personnel	510	1.16	30	Faculty, Medical	182	0.41
11	Surgeons	502	1.14	31	Family Practice	178	0.40
12	Patient Care	419	0.95	32	Orthopedics	174	0.40
13	Education, Medical	359	0.82	33	Learning	173	0.39
14	Simulation Training	357	0.81	34	Ophthalmology	172	0.39
15	Laparoscopy	357	0.81	35	Radiology	149	0.34
16	Pediatrics	311	0.71	36	Surveys and Questionnaires	140	0.32
17	Internal Medicine	298	0.68	37	Physicians, Primary Care	140	0.32
18	Emergency Medicine	262	0.60	38	Certification	133	0.30
19	Computer Simulation	256	0.58	39	Patient Simulation	127	0.29
20	Health Knowledge, Attitudes, Practice	238	0.54	40	Learning Curve	123	0.28

图 11　临床技能与医疗服务 2011—2020 年高频主题词分布

2. 临床技能与医疗服务 2011—2020 年高频主题词聚类（图 12）

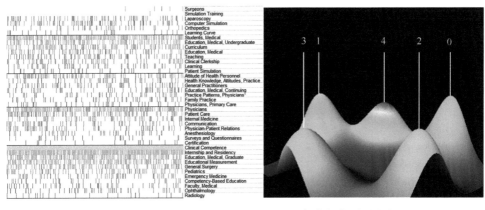

图 12　临床技能与医疗服务 2011—2020 年高频主题词聚类

注：右图中数字表示高频主题词聚类所形成的主题类别

通过高频主题词聚类分析，近 10 年临床技能与医疗服务研究主题涵盖以下 5 个主要方面：

（1）临床技能培训和评估工具的开发与应用。

（2）标准化病人在临床实习期医学生教学与评价中的应用。

（3）对于卫生保健工作者医学知识和临床技能的培训。

（4）医疗服务质量及医患关系影响因素调查。

（5）对住培医师和住院医师临床技能的培训与评价研究。

（三）疾病预防与健康促进

检索策略：Preventive Health Services [MeSH] AND（Physicians [MeSH] OR Internship and Residency [MeSH] OR Students，Medical [MeSH]）。

统计年限：2011 年 1 月 1 日至 2020 年 12 月 31 日。

1. 疾病预防与健康促进 2011—2020 年高频主题词分布（图 13）

序号	主题词	频次	百分比	序号	主题词	频次	百分比
1	Physicians	671	3.79	21	Early Detection of Cancer	114	0.64
2	Attitude of Health Personnel	466	2.63	22	Communication	102	0.58
3	Health Knowledge, Attitudes, Practice	454	2.56	23	Breast Neoplasms	99	0.56
4	Mass Screening	412	2.33	24	Influenza, Human	99	0.56
5	Students, Medical	378	2.14	25	Neoplasms	94	0.53
6	Health Promotion	375	2.12	26	Preventive Health Services	93	0.53
7	Patient Education as Topic	365	2.06	27	Influenza Vaccines	90	0.51
8	General Practitioners	365	2.06	28	Pediatricians	85	0.48
9	Practice Patterns, Physicians'	357	2.02	29	Smoking Cessation	85	0.48
10	Vaccination	305	1.72	30	Health Literacy	83	0.47
11	Physicians, Primary Care	286	1.62	31	Referral and Consultation	82	0.46
12	Primary Health Care	272	1.54	32	Health Personnel	81	0.46
13	Internship and Residency	252	1.42	33	Patient Acceptance of Health Care	79	0.45
14	Physician-Patient Relations	185	1.04	34	Papillomavirus Vaccines	79	0.45
15	Clinical Competence	148	0.84	35	Pediatrics	78	0.44
16	Genetic Testing	137	0.77	36	Counseling	77	0.43
17	Health Education	134	0.76	37	Parents	76	0.43
18	Physicians, Family	122	0.69	38	Surgeons	72	0.41
19	Physician's Role	121	0.68	39	Guideline Adherence	70	0.40
20	HIV Infections	117	0.66	40	Internet	70	0.40

图 13　疾病预防与健康促进 2011—2020 年高频主题词分布

2. 疾病预防与健康促进 2011—2020 年高频主题词聚类（图 14）

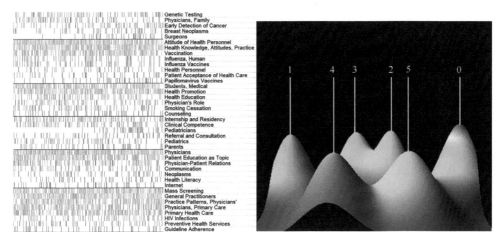

图 14 疾病预防与健康促进 2011—2020 年高频主题词聚类

注：右图中数字表示高频主题词聚类所形成的主题类别

通过高频主题词聚类分析，近 10 年疾病预防与健康促进研究主题涵盖以下 6 个主要方面：

（1）实施癌症早期筛查和制定癌症防治指南。

（2）初级卫生保健工作者对流感疫苗接种接受度的相关调查。

（3）对临床医师和医学生吸烟行为的健康教育与戒烟行动。

（4）基于互联网的健康素养与病人教育。

（5）艾滋病筛查和防治宣传。

（6）其他，包括疫苗安全性培训和免费疫苗计划推广。

（四）信息与管理

检索策略：（Information Management [MeSH] OR Self-Management [MeSH] OR Time Management [MeSH] OR Leadership [MeSH]）AND（Physicians [MeSH] OR Internship and Residency [MeSH] OR Students，Medical [MeSH]）。

统计年限：2011 年 1 月 1 日至 2020 年 12 月 31 日。

1. 信息与管理 2011—2020 年高频主题词分布（图 15）

序号	主题词	频次	百分比	序号	主题词	频次	百分比
1	Physicians	1438	5.52	21	Data Collection	180	0.69
2	Internship and Residency	1066	4.09	22	General Surgery	169	0.65
3	Leadership	864	3.32	23	Communication	162	0.62
4	Students, Medical	810	3.11	24	Curriculum	157	0.60
5	Attitude of Health Personnel	800	3.07	25	Narration	150	0.58
6	General Practitioners	447	1.72	26	Decision-Making	143	0.55
7	Clinical Competence	411	1.58	27	Interprofessional Relations	142	0.55
8	Physicians, Women	294	1.13	28	Personnel Selection	139	0.53
9	Physician-Patient Relations	279	1.07	29	Family Practice	134	0.51
10	Education, Medical, Graduate	277	1.06	30	Physicians, Family	133	0.51
11	Faculty, Medical	255	0.98	31	Pediatrics	130	0.50
12	Health Knowledge, Attitudes, Practice	250	0.96	32	Delivery of Health Care	130	0.50
13	Education, Medical, Undergraduate	245	0.94	33	Patient Care Team	120	0.46
14	Practice Patterns, Physicians'	230	0.88	34	Learning	114	0.44
15	Primary Health Care	227	0.87	35	Teaching	113	0.43
16	Interviews as Topic	226	0.87	36	Schools, Medical	112	0.43
17	Education, Medical	213	0.82	37	Internal Medicine	111	0.43
18	Surgeons	210	0.81	38	Physician's Role	111	0.43
19	Career Choice	196	0.75	39	Educational Measurement	104	0.40
20	Physicians, Primary Care	188	0.72	40	Neoplasms	103	0.40

图 15　信息与管理 2011—2020 年高频主题词分布

2. 信息与管理 2011—2020 年高频主题词聚类（图 16）

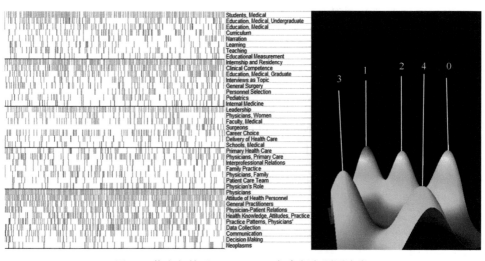

图 16　信息与管理 2011—2020 年高频主题词聚类

注：右图中数字表示高频主题词聚类所形成的主题类别

通过高频主题词聚类分析，近 10 年信息与管理研究主题涵盖以下 5 个主要方面：

（1）叙事医学在医学教育中的应用。

（2）住培医师录取和住院医师招聘的影响因素研究。

（3）性别与领导力的关系研究。

（4）家庭医生在初级卫生保健中扮演的角色。

（5）医师在临床诊疗中如何作出临床决策的研究。

（五）人际沟通

检索策略：Communication [MeSH] AND Interpersonal Relations [MeSH] AND（Physicians [MeSH] OR Internship and Residency [MeSH] OR Students，Medical [MeSH]）。

统计年限：2011 年 1 月 1 日至 2020 年 12 月 31 日。

1. 人际沟通 2011—2020 年高频主题词分布（图 17）

序号	主题词	频次	百分比	序号	主题词	频次	百分比
1	Physician-Patient Relations	1222	6.16	21	Referral and Consultation	134	0.68
2	Communication	1164	5.87	22	Patient Satisfaction	126	0.64
3	Physicians	1120	5.65	23	Patient-Centered Care	125	0.63
4	Students, Medical	466	2.35	24	Conflict of Interest	120	0.61
5	Attitude of Health Personnel	463	2.34	25	Education, Medical	119	0.60
6	Internship and Residency	422	2.13	26	Truth Disclosure	105	0.53
7	Interdisciplinary Communication	392	1.98	27	Practice Patterns, Physicians'	103	0.52
8	Clinical Competence	314	1.58	28	Empathy	103	0.52
9	Disclosure	302	1.52	29	Oncologists	100	0.50
10	Interprofessional Relations	276	1.39	30	Terminal Care	97	0.49
11	General Practitioners	274	1.38	31	Drug Industry	96	0.48
12	Neoplasms	211	1.06	32	Education, Medical, Graduate	96	0.48
13	Patient Care Team	202	1.02	33	Professional-Family Relations	94	0.47
14	Education, Medical, Undergraduate	173	0.87	34	Curriculum	92	0.46
15	Health Knowledge, Attitudes, Practice	164	0.83	35	Communication Barriers	87	0.44
16	Physicians, Primary Care	159	0.80	36	Pediatrics	87	0.44
17	Primary Health Care	154	0.78	37	Physician's Role	84	0.42
18	Decision-Making	146	0.74	38	Patient Participation	84	0.42
19	Surgeons	143	0.72	39	General Surgery	80	0.40
20	Cooperative Behavior	138	0.70	40	Negotiating	80	0.40

图 17　人际沟通 2011—2020 年高频主题词分布

2. 人际沟通 2011—2020 年高频主题词聚类（图 18）

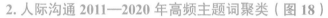

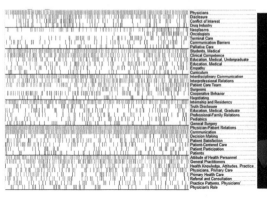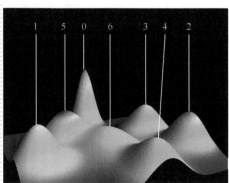

图 18　人际沟通 2011—2020 年高频主题词聚类

注：右图中数字表示高频主题词聚类所形成的主题类别

通过高频主题词聚类分析，近 10 年人际沟通研究主题涵盖以下 7 个主要方面：

（1）揭示医药行业利益冲突的重要举措——阳光法案。

（2）医护人员与癌症病人就临终关怀问题产生的沟通障碍。

（3）隐性课程对医学生临床技能（如与病人互动）和同理心的影响。

（4）临床医师的跨专业交流与合作研究。

（5）临床医师与病人家属的沟通研究和相关沟通技能评价工具的开发与应用。

（6）临床医师的沟通方式与病人参与临床决策的质量的关系研究。

（7）医疗保健提供者在病人健康管理中的作用。

（六）团队合作

检索策略：（Cooperative Behavior [MeSH] OR Patient Care Team [MeSH] OR Intersectoral Collaboration[MeSH] OR Interprofessional Relations[MeSH]）AND（Physicians [MeSH] OR Internship and Residency [MeSH] OR Students，Medical [MeSH]）。

统计年限：2011 年 1 月 1 日至 2020 年 12 月 31 日。

1. 团队合作 2011—2020 年高频主题词分布（图 19）

序号	主题词	频次	百分比	序号	主题词	频次	百分比
1	Interprofessional Relations	1165	4.79	21	Referral and Consultation	136	0.56
2	Physicians	1093	4.50	22	Patient-Centered Care	131	0.54
3	Patient Care Team	943	3.88	23	Pediatrics	124	0.51
4	Internship and Residency	730	3.00	24	Hospitalists	123	0.51
5	Attitude of Health Personnel	636	2.62	25	Practice Patterns, Physicians'	121	0.50
6	Students, Medical	635	2.61	26	Quality Improvement	119	0.49
7	Cooperative Behavior	614	2.53	27	Physician's Role	118	0.49
8	Interdisciplinary Communication	392	1.61	28	Physician-Patient Relations	116	0.48
9	Clinical Competence	355	1.46	29	Delivery of Health Care	116	0.48
10	Primary Health Care	332	1.37	30	Nurses	110	0.45
11	General Practitioners	317	1.30	31	Faculty, Medical	110	0.45
12	Pharmacists	263	1.08	32	Family Practice	110	0.45
13	Education, Medical	230	0.95	33	Patient Safety	110	0.45
14	Communication	217	0.89	34	Leadership	107	0.44
15	Education, Medical, Undergraduate	213	0.88	35	Learning	98	0.40
16	Surgeons	208	0.86	36	Drug Industry	97	0.40
17	Physicians, Primary Care	198	0.81	37	Psychiatry	97	0.40
18	Education, Medical, Graduate	193	0.79	38	Health Personnel	97	0.40
19	General Surgery	160	0.66	39	Health Knowledge, Attitudes, Practice	97	0.40
20	Curriculum	143	0.59	40	Students, Nursing	96	0.39

图 19　团队合作 2011—2020 年高频主题词分布

2. 团队合作 2011—2020 年高频主题词聚类（图 20）

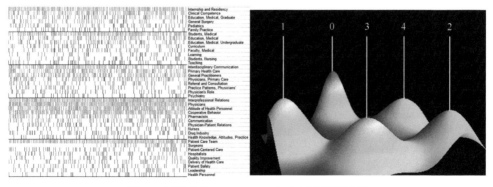

图 20　团队合作 2011—2020 年高频主题词聚类

注：右图中数字表示高频主题词聚类所形成的主题类别

通过高频主题词聚类分析，近 10 年团队合作研究主题涵盖以下 5 个主要方面：

（1）强化初级卫生保健工作者临床技能培训的方法研究。

（2）临床医学学生和护理学生跨专业合作的课程开发与应用。

（3）临床医师与初级卫生保健工作者的跨专业交流与合作研究。

（4）临床医师、护士和药剂师对于跨专业合作的态度研究。

（5）在医疗团队中领导力面临的挑战和机遇。

（七）科学研究

检索策略：Research [MeSH] AND（Physicians [MeSH] OR Internship and Residency [MeSH] OR Students，Medical [MeSH]）。

统计年限：2011 年 1 月 1 日至 2020 年 12 月 31 日。

1. 科学研究 2011—2020 年高频主题词分布（图 21）

序号	主题词	频次	百分比	序号	主题词	频次	百分比
1	Physicians	1500	4.56	21	Faculty, Medical	205	0.62
2	Attitude of Health Personnel	1108	3.37	22	Curriculum	200	0.61
3	Biomedical Research	1099	3.34	23	General Surgery	190	0.58
4	Students, Medical	1081	3.29	24	Research Personnel	185	0.56
5	Internship and Residency	1019	3.10	25	Decision-Making	183	0.56
6	General Practitioners	758	2.30	26	Neoplasms	180	0.55
7	Primary Health Care	493	1.50	27	Physicians, Family	179	0.54
8	Clinical Competence	445	1.35	28	Pediatrics	174	0.53
9	Education, Medical, Undergraduate	385	1.17	29	General Practice	170	0.52
10	Physician-Patient Relations	348	1.06	30	Interprofessional Relations	161	0.49
11	Practice Patterns, Physicians'	322	0.98	31	Learning	153	0.47
12	Education, Medical, Graduate	318	0.97	32	Family Practice	151	0.46
13	Surgeons	302	0.92	33	Research Design	148	0.45
14	Research	278	0.84	34	Qualitative Research	125	0.38
15	Health Knowledge, Attitudes, Practice	268	0.81	35	Nurses	125	0.38
16	Outcome Assessment, Health Care	260	0.79	36	Palliative Care	125	0.38
17	Physicians, Primary Care	257	0.78	37	Referral and Consultation	122	0.37
18	Education, Medical	255	0.78	38	Internal Medicine	120	0.36
19	Career Choice	222	0.67	39	Quality of Health Care	119	0.36
20	Communication	213	0.65	40	Schools, Medical	117	0.36

图 21　科学研究 2011—2020 年高频主题词分布

2. 科学研究 2011—2020 年高频主题词聚类（图 22）

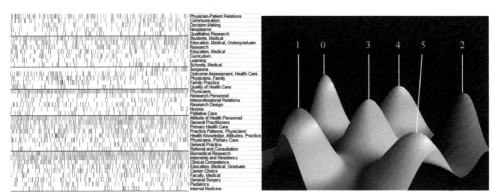

图 22　科学研究 2011—2020 年高频主题词聚类

注：右图中数字表示高频主题词聚类所形成的主题类别

通过高频主题词聚类分析，近 10 年科学研究研究主题涵盖以下 6 个主要方面：

（1）临床医师与重症病人就病情告知问题进行的沟通与决策的研究。

（2）显性课程与隐性课程对医学生（如学习目标、学习结果）的影响研究。

（3）家庭医生对于病人医疗服务质量和结果有效性的研究。

（4）关于医护人员对于姑息治疗的看法与认识的研究。

（5）全科医生对儿童青少年心理问题治疗经验的研究。

（6）执业环境对住培医师学业表现和职业选择的影响研究。

（八）核心价值观与职业素养

检索策略：（Value of Life [MeSH] OR Social Values [MeSH] OR Codes of Ethics [MeSH] AND Ethics，Professional [MeSH] OR Humanism [MeSH] OR Professional Misconduct [MeSH] OR Altruism [MeSH] OR Professionalism[tiab] OR "professional performance*" [tiab] OR "professional behavior*" [tiab] OR "unprofessional behavior*" OR "professional attitude*" [tiab] OR "professional identity formation" [tiab]）AND（Physicians [MeSH] OR Internship and Residency [MeSH] OR Students，Medical [MeSH]）。

统计年限：2011 年 1 月 1 日至 2020 年 12 月 31 日。

1. 核心价值观与职业素养 2011—2020 年高频主题词分布（图 23）

序号	主题词	频次	百分比	序号	主题词	频次	百分比
1	Students, Medical	751	6.65	21	Altruism	79	0.70
2	Physicians	679	6.01	22	Social Media	79	0.70
3	Internship and Residency	672	5.95	23	Physician's Role	78	0.69
4	Clinical Competence	387	3.43	24	Clinical Clerkship	72	0.64
5	Professionalism	287	2.54	25	Teaching	68	0.60
6	General Surgery	287	2.54	26	Interprofessional Relations	63	0.56
7	Professional Misconduct	272	2.41	27	Communication	61	0.54
8	Education, Medical, Under-graduate	268	2.37	28	Career Choice	59	0.52
9	Attitude of Health Personnel	219	1.94	29	Empathy	59	0.52
10	Education, Medical, Graduate	212	1.88	30	Burnout, Professional	56	0.50
11	Physician-Patient Relations	196	1.74	31	Health Knowledge, Attitudes, Practice	54	0.48
12	Education, Medical	184	1.63	32	Orthopedics	52	0.46
13	Curriculum	153	1.35	33	Social Identification	50	0.44
14	Ethics, Medical	149	1.32	34	Pediatrics	50	0.44
15	Professional Competence	138	1.22	35	Practice Patterns, Physicians'	47	0.42
16	Educational Measurement	119	1.05	36	Scientific Misconduct	44	0.39
17	Faculty, Medical	112	0.99	37	Learning	43	0.38
18	Humanism	101	0.89	38	Surveys and Questionnaires	43	0.38
19	Surgeons	88	0.78	39	Delivery of Health Care	42	0.37
20	Schools, Medical	84	0.74	40	General Practitioners	42	0.37

图 23   核心价值观与职业素养 2011—2020 年高频主题词分布

2. 核心价值观与职业素养 2011—2020 年高频主题词聚类（图 24）

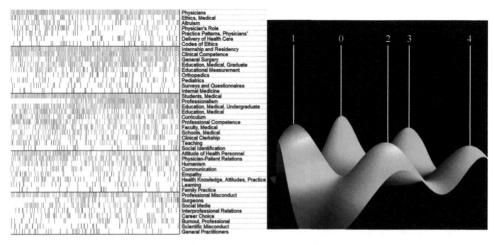

图 24   核心价值观与职业素养 2011—2020 年高频主题词聚类

注：右图中数字表示高频主题词聚类所形成的主题类别

通过高频主题词聚类分析，近 10 年核心价值观与职业素养研究主题涵盖以下 5 个主要方面：

（1）医师角色与医师职业精神的伦理属性。

（2）住培医师职业精神调查工具的开发与应用。

（3）不同文化背景下的医师职业精神及其培养模式。

（4）医学教育研究与实践中的医师职业精神（人道主义、同理心等）。

（5）临床医师的职业不端行为（包括学术不端）研究和职业倦怠现状与应对策略研究。

三、全球医学教育技术研究专题分析

（一）研究方法

1. 检索策略

MeSH 主题词"Education，Medical"＋ JCR 数据库中教育门类下 10 种医学教育期刊（*Academic Medicine / Medical Education / Medical Teacher / BMC Medical Education / Journal of Surgical Education / Advances in Health Sciences Education / Teaching and Learning in Medicine / Medical Education Online / Anatomical Sciences Education / Academic Psychiatry*）AND MeSH 主题词"Educational Technology"。

2. 统计年限

2011 年 1 月 1 日至 2020 年 12 月 31 日。

3. 分析方法

文献概览采用可视化分析工具 CiteSpace 对高发文量国家、机构、作者进行统计；对近 10 年纳入文献（2011—2020）的主要主题词进行高频主题词聚类分析；对 2011—2020 年纳入文献的高被引文献进行共被引聚类分析。

（二）文献概览及研究前沿

1. 全球医学教育技术研究 2011—2020 年发文量国家分布（图 25）

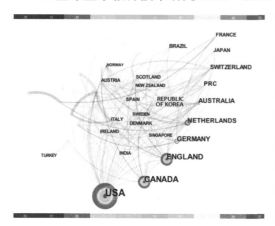

序号	国家 / 地区	发文量	中介中心度
1	USA	721	0.69
2	Canada	183	0.38
3	England	138	0.36
4	Germany	73	0.05
5	Netherlands	62	0.15
6	Australia	60	0.07
7	PRC	49	0.04
8	Switzerland	34	0.05
9	Japan	32	0.00
10	France	31	0.02
11	Brazil	30	0.01
12	Republic of Korea	27	0.03
13	Spain	23	0.02
14	Italy	21	0.03
15	India	21	0.00

图 25　全球医学教育技术研究 2011—2020 年发文量国家分布

注：左图中的 CiteSpace 发文年环代表着文献的发文历史，年环的整体大小反映某个国家的累计发文量。发文年环的颜色代表相应的发文时间。一个年环厚度和相应的时间分区内发文数量成正比。不同国家间的连线表示对应的论文合著关系。引文年环类同。右图中的中介中心度表示一个给定节点在其他节点之间的位置，中心度的值越大表示该节点在网络中越重要，与其他节点的联系（合作）越密切

2. 全球医学教育技术研究 2011—2020 年发文量机构分布（图 26）

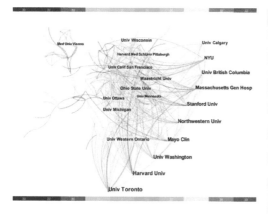

序号	机构	发文量	中介中心度
1	Univ of Toronto	53	0.14
2	Harvard Univ	37	0.07
3	Univ of Washington	32	0.08
4	Mayo Clin	30	0.07
5	Northwestern Univ	29	0.04
6	Stanford Univ	24	0.04
7	Massachusetts Gen Hosp	23	0.03
8	Univ of British Columbia	23	0.02
9	NYU	19	0.07
10	Univ of Calgary	18	0.00
11	Maastricht Univ	17	0.03
12	Univ Western Ontario	16	0.01
13	Univ Wisconsin	15	0.04
14	Ohio State Univ	15	0.01
15	Univ of Michigan	13	0.02

图 26　全球医学教育技术研究 2011—2020 年发文量机构分布

注：左图中的 CiteSpace 可视化高发文量机构分布呈现出不同机构的发文量、发文时间和不同机构间紧密的合作状态

3. 全球医学教育技术研究 2011—2020 年发文量作者分布（图 27）

序号	高发文作者	所在机构	发文量
1	McLaughlin, Kevin	Univ of Calgary	9
2	Fann, James I.	Stanford Univ	8
3	Cook, David A.	Mayo Clin	7
4	Han, David C.	Penn State Univ	7
5	Hatala, Rose	Univ of British Columbia	7
6	Kim, Sara	Univ of Washington	7
7	Miller, Scarlett R.	Penn State Univ	7
8	Moore, Jason Z.	Penn State Univ	7
9	Pepley, David F.	Penn State Univ	7
10	Van der Vleuten, Cees	Maastricht Univ	7
11	Wilson, Timothy D.	Univ of Western Ontario	7
12	Fung, Kevin	Univ of Western Ontario	6
13	Hicks, George L.	Univ of Rochester	6
14	Rossaint, Rolf	Univ of Hosp RWTH Aachen	6
15	Shin, Dong Sun	Ajou Univ	6

图 27 全球医学教育技术研究 2011—2020 年发文量作者分布

注：左图的 CiteSpace 可视化高发文量作者分布呈现出不同作者的发文量、发文时间和不同作者间的相互合作关系

4. 全球医学教育技术研究 2011—2020 年高频主题词分布（图 28）

序号	主题词	频次	百分比	序号	主题词	频次	百分比
1	Clinical Competence	408	4.87	21	Anesthesiology	79	0.94
2	Internship and Residency	368	4.39	22	Patient Simulation	79	0.94
3	Models, Anatomic	350	4.17	23	Curriculum	79	0.94
4	Education, Medical	328	3.91	24	Learning	68	0.81
5	Education, Medical, Undergraduate	258	3.08	25	Audiovisual Aids	67	0.80
6	Education, Medical, Graduate	257	3.07	26	Motion Pictures	65	0.78
7	Manikins	196	2.34	27	Cardiopulmonary Resuscitation	61	0.73
8	Students, Medical	195	2.33	28	Emergency Medicine	57	0.68
9	Simulation Training	184	2.19	29	Intubation, Intratracheal	56	0.67
10	Teaching	165	1.97	30	Laparoscopy	56	0.67
11	Computer Simulation	147	1.75	31	Imaging, Three-Dimensional	52	0.62
12	Computer-Assisted Instruction	114	1.36	32	Psychiatry	44	0.52
13	Educational Technology	108	1.29	33	Communication	44	0.52
14	Educational Measurement	104	1.24	34	Multimedia	41	0.49
15	Anatomy	99	1.18	35	Internet	40	0.48
16	General Surgery	89	1.06	36	Problem-Based Learning	40	0.48
17	Education, Medical, Continuing	87	1.04	37	Otolaryngology	38	0.45
18	Pediatrics	81	0.97	38	Resuscitation	36	0.43
19	Videotape Recording	80	0.95	39	Neurosurgery	34	0.41
20	Printing, Three-Dimensional	79	0.94	40	User-Computer Interface	34	0.41

图 28 全球医学教育技术研究 2011—2020 年高频主题词分布

5. 全球医学教育技术研究 2011—2020 年前 1% 高频被引论文分布（图 29）

序号	高频被引论文	被引频次
1	McGaghie W C, Issenberg S B, Cohen E R, Barsuk J H, Wayne D B. Does simulation-based medical education with deliberate practice yield better results than traditional clinical education? A meta-analytic comparative review of the evidence. Acad Med. 2011 Jun;86(6):706-711.	695
2	French S D, Green S E, O'Connor D A, McKenzie J E, Francis J J, Michie S, Buchbinder R, Schattner P, Spike N, Grimshaw J M. Developing theory-informed behaviour change interventions to implement evidence into practice: a systematic approach using the Theoretical Domains Framework. Implement Sci. 2012 Apr 24;7:38.	523
3	Motola I, Devine L A, Chung H S, Sullivan J E, Issenberg S B. Simulation in healthcare education: a best evidence practical guide. AMEE Guide No. 82. Med Teach. 2013 Oct;35(10):e1511-e1530.	297
4	Andreatta P, Saxton E, Thompson M, Annich G. Simulation-based mock codes significantly correlate with improved pediatric patient cardiopulmonary arrest survival rates. Pediatr Crit Care Med. 2011 Jan;12(1):33-38.	205
5	Hamstra S J, Brydges R, Hatala R, Zendejas B, Cook D A. Reconsidering fidelity in simulation-based training. Acad Med. 2014 Mar;89(3):387-392.	185
6	Preece D, Williams S B, Lam R, Weller R. "Let's get physical": advantages of a physical model over 3D computer models and textbooks in learning imaging anatomy. Anat Sci Educ. 2013 Jul-Aug;6(4):216-224.	174
7	Jaffar A A. YouTube: An emerging tool in anatomy education. Anat Sci Educ. 2012 May-Jun;5(3):158-164.	137
8	Moro C, Štromberga Z, Raikos A, Stirling A. The effectiveness of virtual and augmented reality in health sciences and medical anatomy. Anat Sci Educ. 2017 Nov;10(6):549-559.	133
9	Kogan J R, Conforti L, Bernabeo E, Iobst W, Holmboe E. Opening the black box of clinical skills assessment via observation: a conceptual model. Med Educ. 2011 Oct;45(10):1048-1060.	127
10	Costello J P, Olivieri L J, Su L, Krieger A, Alfares F, Thabit O, Marshall M B, Yoo S J, Kim P C, Jonas R A, Nath D S. Incorporating three-dimensional printing into a simulation-based congenital heart disease and critical care training curriculum for resident physicians. Congenit Heart Dis. 2015 Mar-Apr;10(2):185-190.	107
11	Cannon W D, Garrett W E Jr, Hunter R E, Sweeney H J, Eckhoff D G, Nicandri G T, Hutchinson M R, Johnson D D, Bisson L J, Bedi A, Hill J A, Koh J L, Reinig K D. Improving residency training in arthroscopic knee surgery with use of a virtual-reality simulator. A randomized blinded study. J Bone Joint Surg Am. 2014 Nov 5;96(21):1798-1806.	105
12	Khot Z, Quinlan K, Norman G R, Wainman B. The relative effectiveness of computer-based and traditional resources for education in anatomy. Anat Sci Educ. 2013 Jul-Aug;6(4):211-215.	98
13	Durning S, Artino A R Jr, Pangaro L, van der Vleuten C P, Schuwirth L. Context and clinical reasoning: understanding the perspective of the expert's voice. Med Educ. 2011 Sep;45(9):927-938.	97
14	Hunt E A, Duval-Arnould J M, Nelson-McMillan K L, Bradshaw J H, Diener-West M, Perretta J S, Shilkofski N A. Pediatric resident resuscitation skills improve after "rapid cycle deliberate practice" training. Resuscitation. 2014 Jul;85(7):945-951.	97
15	Diesen D L, Erhunmwunsee L, Bennett K M, Ben-David K, Yurcisin B, Ceppa E P, Omotosho P A, Perez A, Pryor A. Effectiveness of laparoscopic computer simulator versus usage of box trainer for endoscopic surgery training of novices. J Surg Educ. 2011 Jul-Aug;68(4):282-289.	93
16	Davis C R, Bates A S, Ellis H, Roberts A M. Human anatomy: let the students tell us how to teach. Anat Sci Educ. 2014 Jul-Aug;7(4):262-272.	91

图 29　全球医学教育技术研究 2011—2020 年前 1% 高频被引论文分布

6. 全球医学教育技术研究近 10 年（2011—2020）高频主题词聚类（图 30）

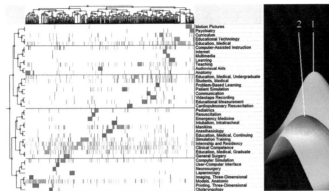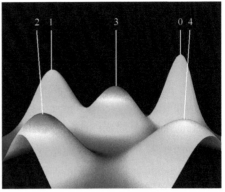

图 30　全球医学教育技术研究 2011—2020 年高频主题词聚类

注：右图中数字表示高频主题词聚类所形成的主题类别

通过高频主题词聚类分析，全球医学教育技术研究主题涵盖以下 5 个主要方面：

（1）数字化信息技术在医学教育研究和教学中的应用。

（2）人体解剖学在线学习资源建设与教学效果评估。

（3）虚拟仿真在医学实验教学和临床教学中的应用。

（4）使用标准化病人培养和评价医学生的沟通能力。

（5）医学模拟训练在毕业后教育临床实践中的应用。

7. 全球医学教育技术研究 2011—2020 年引文共被引聚类（图 31）

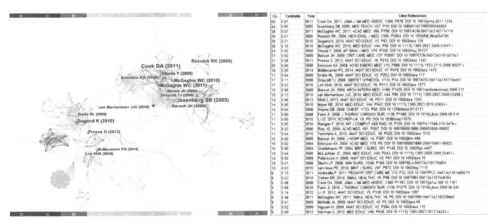

图 31　全球医学教育技术研究 2011—2020 年引文共被引聚类

通过引文共被引聚类分析，近 10 年全球医学教育技术研究高频引文被聚类为以下 7 个主要方面：

（1）3D 打印、三维可视化等教育技术在解剖学教育中的应用。

推荐阅读：

[1] Lim K H, Loo Z Y, Goldie S J, et al. Use of 3D printed models in medical education: A randomized control trial comparing 3D prints versus cadaveric materials for learning external cardiac anatomy. Anat Sci Educ. 2016; 9(3): 213-221.

[2] Yammine K, Violato C. A meta-analysis of the educational effectiveness of three-dimensional visualization technologies in teaching anatomy. Anat Sci Educ. 2015; 8(6): 525-538.

[3] Preece D, Williams S B, Lam R, et al. "Let's get physical": advantages of a physical model over 3D computer models and textbooks in learning imaging anatomy. Anat Sci Educ. 2013; 6(4): 216-224.

[4] Petersson H, Sinkvist D, Wang C, et al. Web-based interactive 3D visualization as a tool for improved anatomy learning. Anat Sci Educ. 2009; 2(2): 61-68.

（2）基于教育技术开发和利用解剖学教学资源。

推荐阅读：

[1] McMenamin P G, Quayle M R, McHenry C R, et al. The production of anatomical teaching resources using three-dimensional (3D) printing technology. Anat Sci Educ. 2014; 7(6): 479-486.

[2] Nguyen N, Wilson T D. A head in virtual reality: development of a dynamic head and neck model. Anat Sci Educ. 2009; 2(6): 294-301.

[3] Khot Z, Quinlan K, Norman G R, et al. The relative effectiveness of computer-based and traditional resources for education in anatomy. Anat Sci Educ. 2013; 6(4): 211-215.

（3）基于互联网的学习对医学教育的影响。

推荐阅读：

[1] Ruiz J G, Mintzer M J, Leipzig R M. The impact of E-learning in medical education. Acad Med. 2006; 81(3): 207-212.

[2] Cook D A, Levinson A J, Garside S, et al. Internet-based learning in the health professions: a meta-analysis. JAMA. 2008; 300(10): 1181-1196.

（4）基于模拟的教育在临床实践中的应用和对医疗质量的影响。

推荐阅读：

[1] McGaghie W C, Issenberg S B, Petrusa E R, et al. A critical review of simulation-based medical education research: 2003-2009. Med Educ. 2010; 44(1): 50-63.

[2] Barsuk J H, McGaghie W C, Cohen E R, et al. Simulation-based mastery learning reduces complications during central venous catheter insertion in a medical intensive care unit. Crit Care Med. 2009; 37(10): 2697-2701.

[3] McGaghie W C, Draycott T J, Dunn W F, et al. Evaluating the impact of simulation on translational patient outcomes. Simul Healthc. 2011; 6 Suppl: 42-47.

[4] Grantcharov T P, Kristiansen V B, Bendix J, et al. Randomized clinical trial of virtual reality simulation for laparoscopic skills training. Br J Surg. 2004; 91(2): 146-150.

（5）模拟逼真度与学习效果的关系研究。

推荐阅读：

[1] Norman G, Dore K, Grierson L. The minimal relationship between simulation fidelity and transfer of learning. Med Educ. 2012; 46(7): 636-647.

[2] Issenberg S B, McGaghie W C, Petrusa E R, et al. Features and uses of high-fidelity medical simulations that lead to effective learning: a BEME systematic review. Med Teach. 2005; 27(1): 10-28.

（6）基于医学模拟的临床技能培训和评价研究。

推荐阅读：

[1] Okuda Y, Bryson E O, DeMaria S Jr, et al. The utility of simulation in medical education: what is the evidence? Mt Sinai J Med. 2009; 76(4): 330-343.

[2] Cook D A, Hatala R, Brydges R, et al. Technology-enhanced simulation for health professions education: a systematic review and meta-analysis. JAMA. 2011; 306(9): 978-988.

[3] Sturm L P, Windsor J A, Cosman P H, et al. A systematic review of skills transfer after surgical simulation training. Ann Surg. 2008; 248(2): 166-179.

（7）医学教育相关理论研究。

推荐阅读：

[1] van Merriënboer J J, Sweller J. Cognitive load theory in health professional education: design principles and strategies. Med Educ. 2010; 44(1): 85-93.

[2] Mayer R E. Applying the science of learning to medical education. Med Educ. 2010; 44(6): 543-549.

四、医学教育学科 ESI 排名

ESI（Essential Science Indicators）基本科学指标数据库，是由国际学术信息数据库公司汤森路透推出的衡量科学研究绩效、跟踪科学发展趋势的基本分析评价工具，是基于 Web of Science 引文索引数据库 Science Citation Index（简称 SCI）和 Social Science Citation Index（简称 SSCI）所收录的全球 8500 多种学术期刊的 1000 多万条文献记录而建立的计量分析数据库。ESI 从引文分析的角度，将全部科学分为 22 个专业领域，分别对国家（地区）、研究机构、期刊、论文以及科学家进行统计分析和排序。ESI 是当今世界范围内普遍用以评价高校、学术机构、国家（地区）国际学术水平及影响力的重要评价指标工具之一。

机构发表论文的总被引量是反映一个机构学术能力和影响力的重要指标之一。建设世界一流大学和一流学科，是中国做出的重大战略决策，有利于提升一个国家高等教育综合实力和国际竞争力。ESI 前百分之一和千分之一的学科及其相应机构是一流学科和一流大学的重要评价指标之一。因此，我们通过与科睿唯安公司合作，将 ESI 排名的概念引入到了医学教育研究领域，为医学教育学科单独建立 ESI 研究机构统计分析和排序。通过介绍医学教育学科 ESI 机构排名的情况，能够发扬优势也寻找差距，可以为未来的研究和实践工作指明方向。

在《2019 国际医学教育研究前沿报告》中我们首次发布了医学教育的 ESI 机构统计排名，受到了广泛好评和欢迎。在 2021 年我们将延续这一内容，将医学教育研究领域 ESI 机构统计排名更新至 2020 年，为全球学者提供更好的参考数据。

（一）研究方法

1. 检索策略

MeSH 主题词"Education，Medical"+ JCR 数据库中教育门类下 10 种医学教育期刊（*Academic Medicine / Medical Education / Medical Teacher / BMC Medical Education / Journal of Surgical Education / Advances in Health Sciences Education / Teaching and Learning in Medicine / Medical Education Online / Anatomical Sciences Education / Academic Psychiatry*）。

2. 统计年限

2011 年 1 月 1 日至 2020 年 12 月 31 日。

3. 统计方法

对纳入检索范围论文的总被引用频次进行统计，通过总被引频次反映学术影响力。

（二）医学教育学科 ESI 机构分布

1. ESI 前 1‰ 机构分布（22/22083）（图 32）

序号	ESI 前 1‰机构	所属国家	10 年累计被引量（2011-2020）	10 年累计发文量（2011-2020）	10 年平均被引量（2011-2020）
1	Univ of Toronto	Canada	15692	1478	10.62
2	Mayo Clin	USA	12293	975	12.61
3	Harvard Univ	USA	11207	894	12.54
4	Univ of Calif San Francisco	USA	10213	1137	8.98
5	Maastricht Univ	Netherlands	7967	717	11.11
6	Univ of Michigan	USA	7868	976	8.06
7	Univ of British Columbia	Canada	7798	659	11.83
8	Northwestern Univ	USA	7409	695	10.66
9	Univ of Penn	USA	7201	862	8.35
10	Univ of Ottawa	Canada	7079	574	12.33
11	Univ of Washington	USA	7066	830	8.51
12	Stanford Univ	USA	6916	778	8.89
13	Johns Hopkins Univ	USA	5830	706	8.26
14	Yale Univ	USA	5617	541	10.38
15	McGill Univ	Canada	5432	532	10.21
16	Massachusetts Gen Hosp	USA	5358	639	8.38
17	McMaster Univ	Canada	5247	555	9.45
18	Duke Univ	USA	5104	574	8.89
19	Brigham & Womens Hosp	USA	5044	556	9.07
20	Vanderbilt Univ	USA	4844	550	8.81
21	Univ of Calgary	Canada	4548	496	9.17
22	Oregon Hlth & Sci Univ	USA	4306	505	8.53

图 32　ESI 前 1‰ 机构分布

2. 各大洲 ESI 排名前 5 机构分布（图 33）

所属大洲	序号	ESI排名	是否进入ESI前1%	机构	所属国家	10年累计被引量（2011-2020）	10年累计发文量（2011-2020）	10年平均被引量（2011-2020）
北美洲	1	1	√	Univ of Toronto	Canada	15692	1478	10.62
	2	2	√	Mayo Clin	USA	12293	975	12.61
	3	3	√	Harvard Univ	USA	11207	894	12.54
	4	4	√	Univ of Calif San Francisco	USA	10213	1137	8.98
	5	6	√	Univ of Michigan	USA	7868	976	8.06
欧洲	1	5	√	Maastricht Univ	Netherlands	7966	716	11.13
	2	31	√	Univ of Dundee	UK	3642	200	18.21
	3	40	√	Univ of London Imperial Coll Sci Technol & Med	UK	3205	263	12.19
	4	54	√	Univ of Glasgow	UK	2502	103	24.29
	5	55	√	Univ of Med Ctr Utrecht	Netherlands	2464	203	12.14
大洋洲	1	39	√	Univ of Melbourne	Australia	3210	335	9.58
	2	41	√	Univ of Sydney	Australia	3155	367	8.60
	3	43	√	Monash Univ	Australia	2908	390	7.46
	4	73	√	Flinders Univ of S Australia	Australia	1979	196	10.10
	5	75	√	Univ of Queensland	Australia	1960	236	8.31
亚洲	1	132	√	King Saud Univ	Saudi Arabia	1073	138	7.78
	2	162	√	Natl Univ of Singapore	Singapore	860	153	5.62
	3	220	√	Univ of Hong Kong	PRC	634	80	7.93
	4	258		Yonsei Univ	Republic of Korea	514	38	13.53
	5	287		Nanyang Technol Univ	Singapore	462	52	8.88
非洲	1	125	√	Univ of Cape Town	South Africa	1111	102	10.89
	2	218	√	Univ of Stellenbosch	South Africa	636	57	11.16
	3	329		Univ of Malawi	Malawi	378	33	11.45
	4	393		Univ of KwaZula-Natal	South Africa	312	61	5.11
	5	432		Univ of Ibadan	Nigeria	288	22	13.09
南美洲	1	213	√	Univ of Sao Paulo	Brazil	664	137	4.85
	2	357		Pontificia Univ of Catolica Chile	Chile	347	90	3.86
	3	430		Univ of Fed Sao Paulo	Brazil	288	45	6.40
	4	458		Hosp Clin Porto Alegre	Brazil	268	5	53.60
	5	654		Univ of Fed Uberlandia	Brazil	177	12	14.75

图 33　各大洲 ESI 排名前 5 机构分布

3. 中国 ESI 排名前 20 机构分布（图 34）

序号	ESI 排名	是否进入ESI前1%	机构	10年累计被引量（2011-2020）	10年累计发文量（2011-2020）	10年平均被引量（2011-2020）
1	220	√	Univ of Hong Kong	634	80	7.93
2	375		Taiwan Univ	326	60	5.43
3	428		Chinese Univ of Hong Kong	289	43	6.72
4	450		Sichuan Univ	273	36	7.58
5	452		Peking Univ	271	58	4.67
6	581		Chang Gung Univ	203	61	3.33
7	676		Yang Ming Univ	171	47	3.64
8	712		I Shou Univ	163	14	11.64
9	867		China Med Univ	130	33	3.94
10	883		Sun Yat-sen Univ	127	35	3.63
11	883		Third Mil Med Univ	127	35	3.63
12	902		Zhejiang Univ	123	15	8.20
13	1008		Capital Med Univ	110	26	4.23
14	1068		Shanghai Jiao Tong Univ	103	31	3.32
15	1134		Fudan Univ	95	42	2.26
16	1242		Central South Univ	86	23	3.74
17	1315		Fourth Mil Med Univ	80	12	6.67
18	1390		Taipei Med Univ	75	38	1.97
19	1505		Hong Kong Polytech Univ	68	11	6.18
20	1563		Chinese Acad Med Sci	65	30	2.17

图 34　中国 ESI 排名前 20 机构分布

五、医学教育研究期刊解析

（一）研究方法

在 JCR 数据库教育门类下的全部期刊中（包括 SCIE 收录期刊 41 种和 SSCI 收录期刊 243 种）按照纳入标准筛选出医学教育研究期刊。

纳入标准：如果某期刊近 10 年来（2010 年 1 月 1 日至 2019 年 12 月 31 日）所发表的期刊论文在 PubMed 数据库中被标引包含 "Education，Medical" [MeSH] 的比例超过 50%，则认为该期刊属于医学教育研究期刊，并将其纳入分析范围。

研究方法：利用书目共现分析系统 Bicomb 统计近 5 年来（2016 年 1 月 1 日至 2020 年 12 月 31 日）全部医学教育研究期刊的高频主题词分布，用来反映该期刊的研究内容与特色主题。

（二）医学教育研究期刊总体概况（图 35）

序号	期刊名称	所属数据库	2020 年中科院期刊分区*（升级版）	影响因子（2019）	主办国家	10 年累计发文量（2011-2020）	被标引为"Education, Medical"[MeSH] 的论文数量	被标引为"Education, Medical"[MeSH]的论文比例（%）
1	Academic Medicine	SCIE	1 区	5.354	USA	4676	2626	56.16
2	Medical Education	SCIE	1 区	4.570	UK	2510	1741	69.36
3	Anatomical Sciences Education	SCIE	2 区	3.759	USA	680	360	52.94
4	Medical Teacher	SCIE	2 区	2.654	UK	3144	1927	61.29
5	Advances in Health Sciences Education	SCIE/SSCI	2 区	2.480	USA	766	388	50.65
6	Journal of Surgical Education	SCIE	3 区	2.220	USA	1823	1359	74.55
7	Medical Education Online	SSCI	3 区	1.970	UK	514	355	69.07
8	Teaching and Learning in Medicine	SCIE	3 区	1.848	USA	569	380	66.78
9	BMC Medical Education	SCIE/SSCI	3 区	1.831	UK	2417	1399	57.88
10	Academic Psychiatry	SSCI	4 区	2.148	USA	1563	959	61.36

*SCIE- 学科教育类 /SSCI- 教育学和教育研究

图 35 医学 教育研究期刊总体概况

（三）医学教育学科期刊高频主题词分布

1. *Academic Medicine*（图 36）

序号	主题词	频次	百分比	A/O	序号	主题词	频次	百分比	A/O
1	Education, Medical	462	5.27	1.50	16	Attitude of Health Personnel	83	0.95	0.99
2	Students, Medical	438	4.99	1.30	17	Internal Medicine	77	0.88	1.66
3	Internship and Residency	338	3.85	0.55	18	Competency-Based Education	74	0.84	2.52
4	Education, Medical, Undergraduate	269	3.07	1.09	19	Biomedical Research	71	0.81	1.83
5	Curriculum	265	3.02	1.48	20	School Admission Criteria	65	0.74	2.82
6	Clinical Competence	237	2.70	0.75	21	Leadership	62	0.71	2.58
7	Faculty, Medical	200	2.28	2.67	22	Quality Improvement	59	0.67	1.59
8	Schools, Medical	195	2.22	3.05	23	Learning	58	0.66	0.89
9	Education, Medical, Graduate	191	2.18	0.66	24	Licensure, Medical	57	0.65	7.09
10	Physicians	178	2.03	1.61	25	Health Personnel	50	0.57	0.77
11	Educational Measurement	177	2.02	1.58	26	Health Occupations	50	0.57	3.18
12	Physician-Patient Relations	110	1.25	2.60	27	Interprofessional Relations	48	0.55	1.48
13	Academic Medical Centers	102	1.16	5.82	28	Teaching	47	0.54	0.64
14	Delivery of Health Care	94	1.07	0.23	29	Burnout, Professional	45	0.51	1.16
15	Clinical Clerkship	85	0.97	1.96	30	Empathy	45	0.51	1.99

图 36 *Academic Medicine* 高频主题词分布

注：A 表示相应主题词在本期刊所发表的全部论文中所占的比例；O 表示相应主题词在 PubMed 数据库中被标引为 "Education，Medical" [MeSH] 的全部期刊论文中所占的比例；A/O 用来衡量该期刊相应主题词所代表的研究内容的发表倾向程度，其值越大，表示该期刊发表关于相应主题词所代表的研究内容的比例越大，可以为医学教育研究者选择投稿期刊提供参考性意见。（红色字体为 A/O 大于 5 的主题词，为重点关注内容，下同）

2. *Medical Education*（图 37）

序号	主题词	频次	百分比	A/O	序号	主题词	频次	百分比	A/O
1	Education, Medical	233	6.52	1.86	16	Feedback	34	0.95	6.10
2	Students, Medical	231	6.46	1.68	17	Interprofessional Relations	34	0.95	2.56
3	Learning	130	3.64	4.89	18	Schools, Medical	31	0.87	1.19
4	Clinical Competence	129	3.61	1.01	19	Empathy	28	0.78	3.04
5	Internship and Residency	108	3.02	0.43	20	Physician-Patient Relations	26	0.73	1.52
6	Teaching	75	2.10	2.47	21	Simulation Training	26	0.73	0.74
7	Educational Measurement	72	2.01	1.57	22	Workplace	24	0.67	5.39
8	Physicians	66	1.85	1.47	23	Competency-Based Education	23	0.64	1.92
9	Curriculum	65	1.82	0.89	24	Health Personnel	22	0.62	1.50
10	Education, Medical, Undergraduate	65	1.82	0.65	25	Career Choice	22	0.62	0.87
11	Communication	46	1.29	2.66	26	School Admission Criteria	21	0.59	2.25
12	Faculty, Medical	45	1.26	1.48	27	Cooperative Behavior	21	0.59	3.78
13	Problem-Based Learning	41	1.15	2.31	28	Education, Medical, Graduate	21	0.59	0.18
14	Clinical Clerkship	39	1.09	2.20	29	Attitude of Health Personnel	20	0.56	0.58
15	Health Occupations	37	1.03	5.74	30	Medicine	20	0.56	3.82

图 37 *Medical Education* 高频主题词分布

3. *Anatomical Sciences Education*（图 38）

序号	主题词	频次	百分比	A/O	序号	主题词	频次	百分比	A/O
1	Anatomy	259	17.72	39.13	16	Schools, Medical	16	1.09	0.12
2	Education, Medical, Undergraduate	128	8.76	2.30	17	Tissue and Organ Procurement	16	1.09	24.09
3	Students, Medical	108	7.39	0.10	18	Histology	13	0.89	43.21
4	Teaching	44	3.01	3.54	19	Imaging, Three-Dimensional	13	0.89	14.25
5	Learning	41	2.80	3.76	20	Anatomists	13	0.89	21.26
6	Computer-Assisted Instruction	41	2.80	7.67	21	Neuroanatomy	13	0.89	21.71
7	Dissection	33	2.26	24.58	22	Education, Distance	12	0.82	2.46
8	Curriculum	31	2.12	1.04	23	Social Media	11	0.75	3.88
9	Educational Measurement	31	2.12	1.66	24	Health Occupations	11	0.75	4.18
10	Problem-Based Learning	25	1.71	3.43	25	Academic Performance	10	0.68	5.49
11	Students, Health Occupations	23	1.57	11.14	26	Pneumonia, Viral	9	0.62	0.22
12	Cadaver	19	1.30	21.39	27	Coronavirus Infections	9	0.62	0.22
13	Education, Medical	17	1.16	0.33	28	Anatomy, Regional	9	0.62	8.68
14	Models, Anatomic	17	1.16	7.44	29	Printing, Three-Dimensional	9	0.62	6.58
15	Education, Professional	16	1.09	1.23	30	Pandemics	8	0.55	0.28

图 38 *Anatomical Sciences Education* 高频主题词分布

4. *Medical Teacher*（图 39）

序号	主题词	频次	百分比	A/O	序号	主题词	频次	百分比	A/O
1	Students, Medical	396	9.64	2.50	16	Attitude of Health Personnel	46	1.12	1.17
2	Education, Medical	331	8.06	0.02	17	Problem-Based Learning	42	1.02	2.05
3	Education, Medical, Undergraduate	262	6.38	2.27	18	Clinical Clerkship	38	0.93	1.88
4	Educational Measurement	150	3.65	2.86	19	Health Occupations	32	0.78	4.35
5	Clinical Competence	146	3.56	0.99	20	Simulation Training	30	0.73	0.74
6	Learning	121	2.95	3.96	21	Education, Medical, Graduate	30	0.73	0.22
7	Curriculum	99	2.41	1.18	22	Empathy	29	0.71	2.77
8	Faculty, Medical	92	2.24	2.63	23	Formative Feedback	26	0.63	3.95
9	Teaching	84	2.05	2.41	24	Physician-Patient Relations	24	0.58	1.21
10	Schools, Medical	79	1.92	2.63	25	School Admission Criteria	24	0.58	2.21
11	Internship and Residency	69	1.68	0.24	26	Models, Educational	22	0.54	2.99
12	Physicians	55	1.34	1.06	27	Cooperative Behavior	22	0.54	3.46
13	Interprofessional Relations	52	1.27	3.42	28	Professionalism	22	0.54	2.53
14	Competency-Based Education	46	1.12	0.36	29	Peer Group	22	0.54	2.06
15	Health Personnel	46	1.12	2.72	30	Professional Competence	20	0.49	2.43

图 39 *Medical Teacher* 高频主题词分布

5. *Advances in Health Sciences Education*（图 40）

序号	主题词	频次	百分比	A/O	序号	主题词	频次	百分比	A/O
1	Students, Medical	63	5.52	1.43	16	Workplace	15	1.31	10.54
2	Educational Measurement	51	4.47	3.50	17	Faculty, Medical	14	1.23	1.45
3	Education, Medical	46	4.03	1.15	18	Curriculum	14	1.23	0.60
4	Clinical Competence	41	3.59	1.00	19	Clinical Decision-Making	13	1.14	7.44
5	Education, Medical, Undergraduate	41	3.59	1.28	20	Formative Feedback	11	0.96	6.02
6	Schools, Medical	30	2.63	3.61	21	Cognition	10	0.88	10.76
7	School Admission Criteria	27	2.37	9.02	22	Motivation	9	0.79	6.86
8	Learning	25	2.19	2.94	23	Students, Health Occupations	9	0.79	5.61
9	Problem-Based Learning	24	2.10	4.21	24	Physician-Patient Relations	9	0.79	1.64
10	Health Occupations	21	1.84	13.06	25	Attitude of Health Personnel	9	0.79	0.83
11	Education, Medical, Graduate	18	1.58	0.48	26	Models, Educational	8	0.70	3.87
12	Health Personnel	16	1.40	3.39	27	Career Choice	8	0.70	0.98
13	Teaching	16	1.40	1.65	28	Patient Care Team	8	0.70	3.85
14	Physicians	16	1.40	1.11	29	Research	8	0.70	5.53
15	Internship and Residency	16	1.40	0.20	30	College Admission Test	8	0.70	15.31

图 40 *Advances in Health Sciences Education* 高频主题词分布

6. *Journal of Surgical Education*（图 41）

序号	主题词	频次	百分比	A/O	序号	主题词	频次	百分比	A/O
1	General Surgery	388	9.47	8.27	16	Clinical Clerkship	32	0.78	1.57
2	Clinical Competence	371	9.05	2.52	17	Video Recording	31	0.76	5.03
3	Internship and Residency	326	7.96	1.14	18	Personnel Selection	30	0.73	2.75
4	Education, Medical, Graduate	267	6.52	1.98	19	Surgery, Plastic	29	0.71	3.11
5	Simulation Training	138	3.37	3.41	20	Faculty, Medical	28	0.68	0.80
6	Education, Medical, Undergraduate	85	2.07	0.74	21	Patient Care Team	27	0.66	2.54
7	Orthopedics	67	1.63	4.28	22	Quality Improvement	26	0.63	1.50
8	Educational Measurement	65	1.59	1.25	23	Orthopedic Procedures	26	0.63	5.31
9	Curriculum	60	1.46	0.72	24	Competency-Based Education	25	0.61	1.83
10	Laparoscopy	55	1.34	5.02	25	Accreditation	25	0.61	2.96
11	Specialties, Surgical	48	1.17	5.87	26	Robotic Surgical Procedures	24	0.59	3.71
12	Students, Medical	42	1.02	0.26	27	Workload	22	0.54	2.59
13	Surgeons	39	0.95	1.77	28	Biomedical Research	22	0.54	1.22
14	Career Choice	39	0.95	1.33	29	Suture Techniques	21	0.51	7.04
15	Surveys and Questionnaires	34	0.83	3.05	30	Communication	20	0.49	1.01

图 41 *Journal of Surgical Education* 高频主题词分布

7. *Medical Education Online*（图 42）

序号	主题词	频次	百分比	A/O	序号	主题词	频次	百分比	A/O
1	Students, Medical	110	9.23	2.40	16	Learning	13	1.09	1.46
2	Education, Medical, Undergraduate	79	6.63	2.36	17	Education, Distance	13	1.09	3.28
3	Education, Medical	66	5.54	1.58	18	Communication	11	0.92	1.90
4	Internship and Residency	52	4.36	0.62	19	School Admission Criteria	11	0.92	3.50
5	Educational Measurement	36	3.02	2.37	20	Stress, Psychological	10	0.84	4.14
6	Clinical Competence	31	2.60	0.72	21	Interprofessional Relations	9	0.76	2.05
7	Schools, Medical	29	2.43	3.33	22	Pediatrics	9	0.76	1.04
8	Clinical Clerkship	23	1.93	3.89	23	Career Choice	9	0.76	1.06
9	Faculty, Medical	20	1.68	1.98	24	Attitude of Health Personnel	9	0.76	0.79
10	Teaching	20	1.68	1.98	25	Biomedical Research	8	0.67	1.51
11	Problem-Based Learning	19	1.59	3.19	26	Social Media	8	0.67	3.47
12	Pneumonia, Viral	16	1.34	0.47	27	Internal Medicine	8	0.67	1.26
13	Curriculum	16	1.34	0.66	28	Physicians	8	0.67	0.53
14	Coronavirus Infections	15	1.26	0.44	29	Staff Development	7	0.59	4.44
15	Education, Medical, Graduate	14	1.17	0.36	30	Computer-Assisted Instruction	7	0.59	1.62

图 42 *Medical Education Online* 高频主题词分布

8. *Teaching and Learning in Medicine*（图 43）

序号	主题词	频次	百分比	A/O	序号	主题词	频次	百分比	A/O
1	Students, Medical	83	9.79	2.54	16	Preceptorship	9	1.06	14.18
2	Education, Medical, Undergraduate	43	5.07	1.80	17	Problem-Based Learning	9	1.06	2.13
3	Clinical Competence	33	3.89	1.08	18	Teaching	9	1.06	1.25
4	Educational Measurement	29	3.42	2.68	19	Pediatrics	8	0.94	1.29
5	Internship and Residency	27	3.18	0.45	20	Empathy	8	0.94	3.67
6	Education, Medical	27	3.18	0.91	21	Interprofessional Relations	8	0.94	2.53
7	Curriculum	25	2.95	1.45	22	Career Choice	7	0.83	1.16
8	Education, Medical, Graduate	18	2.12	0.64	23	Attitude of Health Personnel	7	0.83	0.87
9	Clinical Clerkship	18	2.12	4.27	24	Quality Improvement	7	0.83	1.97
10	Learning	16	1.89	2.54	25	Health Personnel	6	0.71	1.72
11	Faculty, Medical	15	1.77	2.08	26	Physicians	6	0.71	0.56
12	Internal Medicine	15	1.77	3.33	27	Competency-Based Education	6	0.71	2.13
13	Peer Group	13	1.53	8.67	28	Adaptation, Psychological	6	0.71	10.28
14	Schools, Medical	10	1.18	1.62	29	Group Processes	6	0.71	10.16
15	Professionalism	9	1.06	4.97	30	Formative Feedback	6	0.71	4.45

图 43　*Teaching and Learning in Medicine* 高频主题词分布

9. *BMC Medical Education*（图 44）

序号	主题词	频次	百分比	A/O	序号	主题词	频次	百分比	A/O
1	Students, Medical	609	8.55	2.22	16	Students, Health Occupations	60	0.84	5.96
2	Education, Medical, Undergraduate	371	5.21	1.85	17	Faculty, Medical	59	0.83	0.98
3	Clinical Competence	329	4.62	1.29	18	Computer-Assisted Instruction	58	0.81	2.22
4	Internship and Residency	169	2.37	0.34	19	Health Personnel	56	0.79	1.92
5	Curriculum	156	2.19	1.07	20	Education, Medical, Continuing	53	0.74	0.72
6	Educational Measurement	149	2.09	1.65	21	Professional Competence	50	0.70	3.47
7	Education, Medical	136	1.91	0.54	22	Clinical Clerkship	49	0.69	1.39
8	Attitude of Health Personnel	122	1.71	1.79	23	Communication	48	0.67	1.38
9	Problem-Based Learning	110	1.54	3.09	24	Simulation Training	47	0.66	0.67
10	Schools, Medical	106	1.49	2.04	25	Students, Nursing	47	0.66	5.99
11	Education, Medical, Graduate	103	1.45	0.44	26	Empathy	42	0.59	2.30
12	Teaching	92	1.29	1.52	27	Internal Medicine	41	0.58	1.09
13	Learning	91	1.28	1.72	28	Interprofessional Relations	41	0.58	1.56
14	Physicians	89	1.25	0.99	29	School Admission Criteria	39	0.55	2.09
15	Career Choice	69	0.97	1.36	30	Health Occupations	38	0.53	2.95

图 44　*BMC Medical Education* 高频主题词分布

10. *Academic Psychiatry*（图 45）

序号	主题词	频次	百分比	A/O	序号	主题词	频次	百分比	A/O
1	Psychiatry	477	13.70	20.04	16	Fellowships and Scholarships	33	0.95	1.67
2	Internship and Residency	281	8.07	1.15	17	Teaching	33	0.95	1.12
3	Students, Medical	151	4.34	1.13	18	Education, Medical, Undergraduate	31	0.89	0.32
4	Curriculum	106	3.05	1.50	19	Career Choice	30	0.86	1.20
5	Clinical Competence	67	1.92	0.53	20	Mental Health Services	27	0.78	12.41
6	Attitude of Health Personnel	57	1.64	1.71	21	Substance-Related Disorders	23	0.66	10.52
7	Physicians	56	1.61	1.28	22	Psychotherapy	23	0.66	12.95
8	Mental Disorders	52	1.49	13.73	23	Depression	22	0.63	6.65
9	Education, Medical, Graduate	52	1.49	0.45	24	Stress, Psychological	21	0.60	2.96
10	Faculty, Medical	50	1.44	1.69	25	Social Stigma	21	0.60	11.89
11	Mental Health	47	1.35	11.48	26	Empathy	21	0.60	2.34
12	Clinical Clerkship	47	1.35	2.72	27	Mentors	20	0.57	2.56
13	Education, Medical	45	1.29	0.37	28	Primary Health Care	20	0.57	1.80
14	Burnout, Professional	43	1.24	2.82	29	Child Psychiatry	19	0.55	13.37
15	Health Knowledge, Attitudes, Practice	34	0.98	2.30	30	Global Health	17	0.49	2.72

图 45 *Academic Psychiatry* 高频主题词分布

结　语

2020 年，我们迎来了"国际医学教育研究前沿报告"发布的第四个年头，通过 ESI、医学教育学科期刊解析、临床医师岗位胜任力前沿分析和全球医学教育技术研究专题系列的引入，让这个新生而富有活力的系列报告更加具有权威性和富有特色；通过文献概览及前沿追踪的方式，让我们紧跟医学教育发展的步伐，促进国内外医学高等院校在医学教育方面的交流与合作，研究与创新，携手推动医学教育的发展。

2021 International Medical Education Research Fronts Report

（English Version）

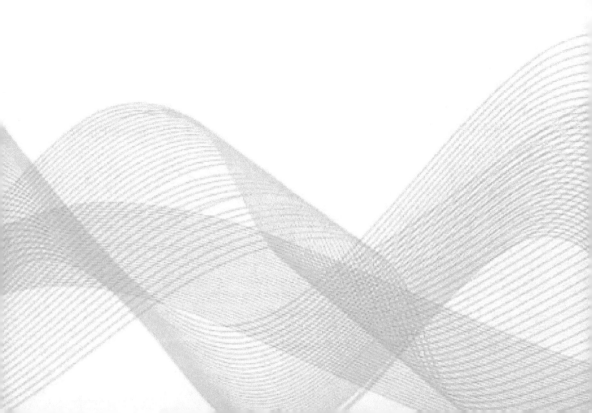

Background

With the acceleration of the internationalization of medical education, current research trends call for mutual learning, timely updates of relevant concepts, understanding of present development trends, and continuous exploration for the future of medical education research and reforms. For three consecutive years, between 2018 and 2020, we released a series of reports on international medical education fronts. We were greatly encouraged by the compelling responses we received from our readers. For 2021, we conducted a systematic analysis of research fronts of Doctor's Common Competency and performed a thematic analysis of medical education technology based on content from previous versions of the report. We hope that this would help medical education researchers and medical educators around the world stay up-to date with current trends in medical education, understand the overall development trends of international medical education, and plan for the future development of medical education research.

Objectives

(1) To comprehensively summarize the current development of global medical education in 2019 and 2020.

(2) To explore research fronts of eight essential factors of doctor's common competency.

(3) To provide reference for the new round of medical education reform by analyzing the progress and trending topics of medical education technology at a global level.

(4) To build the essential science indicators (ESI) ranking for medical education disciplines.

(5) To use bibliometrics to analyze journals in medical education disciplines and to provide reference for medical education researchers when selecting journals for article submission.

Methods

Data collection

Existing literature in the PubMed database was retrieved using the search term: "Education, Medical [MeSH]". The PMID of retrieved articles was matched with the literature retrieved from the Web of Science database (including SCIE and SSCI), and full bibliographic records（including the reference index for each article）were downloaded.

The scope of literature

Based on the data collection, as well as the information and classification of bibliography presented in the Web of Science database, scientometric software packages HistCite and CiteSpace were used to statistically analyze the following indices in the literature: number of publications per country/region, number of citations per country/region, number of publications per institution, number of citations per institution, number of publications per author, number of citations per author, number of publications per journal, and number of citations per journal.

Research fronts

1. Distribution and clustering of high frequent MeSH terms

Based on data collection, BICOMB（Bibliographic Items Co-occurrence Matrix Builder）was used to extract the main MeSH terms from the included literature. After eliminating characteristic MeSH terms that may apply to all studies or results, high frequent MeSH terms were counted and a list of high frequent MeSH terms was generated. A clustering toolkit（gCLUTO）was used to carry out clustering analysis by importing the generated high frequent MeSH terms matrix.

2. Co-citation clustering of references

Co-citation clustering reflects the degree of aggregation among cited articles by analyzing citation relationships. Using BICOMB and gCLUTO, we extracted and ranked the cited articles and generated a co-citation matrix from the included literature for co-citation clustering.

Results

I. Scope of literature and research fronts of medical education research

Search Strategy："Education, Medical [MeSH]" OR（*Academic Medicine / Medical Education / Medical Teacher / BMC Medical Education / Journal of Surgical Education / Advances in Health Sciences Education / Teaching and Learning in Medicine / Medical Education Online / Anatomical Sciences Education / Academic Psychiatry*）[Journal].

Time Range: Since there is a delay in indexing of the most recently published literature by Web of Science, the total number of indexed articles of the current year often does not represent the total number of papers published this year. Therefore, we would need to supplement with the number of papers published in the previous year for literature scope analysis. In this case, the first part of the literature scope analysis for international medical education research included literature from both 2019 and 2020 in order to analyze the current development of global medical education. Additionally, literature published in 2019 were not all included in the 2020 International Medical Education Research Fronts Report due to the delay in indexing by Web of Science, so this method has been used to supplement the missing articles from each previous year of the report.

1. Countries/regions with the most publications and citations related to medical education in 2019 and 2020 (Figure 1)

Ranking	Country/Region	Number of publications	Percentage	Ranking	Country/Region	Number of citations	Percentage	Average number of citations
1	USA	6531	54.88	1	USA	14726	40.12	2.25
2	UK	1352	11.36	2	UK	3133	8.54	2.32
3	Canada	1141	9.59	3	Canada	3043	8.29	2.67
4	Australia	639	5.37	4	Netherlands	1836	5	3.57
5	Netherlands	514	4.32	5	Australia	1759	4.79	2.75
6	Germany	451	3.79	6	Germany	1192	3.25	2.64
7	PRC	359	3.02	7	Italy	827	2.25	4.07
8	France	217	1.82	8	PRC	746	2.03	2.08
9	Italy	203	1.71	9	France	595	1.62	2.74
10	Switzerland	167	1.40	10	Singapore	556	1.51	4.09
11	India	164	1.38	11	Spain	460	1.25	3.13
12	Brazil	162	1.36	12	Sweden	444	1.21	4.58
13	Spain	147	1.24	13	Belgium	426	1.16	4.95
14	Singapore	136	1.14	14	Ireland	409	1.11	3.53
15	Japan	128	1.08	15	New Zealand	389	1.06	3.60

Figure 1　Countries/regions with the most publications and citations related to medical education in 2019 and 2020

2. Institutions with the most publications and citations related to medical education in 2019 and 2020（Figure 2）

Ranking	Institution	Number of publications	Percentage
1	Harvard Med Sch	455	3.82
2	Univ of Toronto	342	2.87
3	Univ of Calif San Francisco	335	2.82
4	Univ of Michigan	305	2.56
5	Mayo Clin	261	2.19
6	Stanford Univ	261	2.19
7	Univ of Penn	221	1.86
8	Univ of Washington	220	1.85
9	Johns Hopkins Univ	203	1.71
10	Maastricht Univ	190	1.60
11	Massachusetts Gen Hosp	187	1.57
12	Northwestern Univ	183	1.54
13	Univ of British Columbia	165	1.39
14	Brigham & Women's Hosp	152	1.28
15	Duke Univ	151	1.27

Ranking	Institution	Number of citations	Percentage	Average number of citations
1	Harvard Med Sch	1320	1.51	2.90
2	Univ of Calif San Francisco	1209	1.39	3.61
3	Univ of Michigan	948	1.09	3.11
4	Univ of Penn	946	1.09	4.28
5	Univ of Toronto	928	1.06	2.71
6	Mayo Clin	911	1.05	3.49
7	Univ of Washington	824	0.95	3.75
8	Northwestern Univ	807	0.93	4.41
9	Stanford Univ	793	0.91	3.04
10	Uniformed Serv Univ of Hlth Sci	609	0.7	4.17
11	Maastricht Univ	607	0.7	3.19
12	Johns Hopkins Univ	587	0.67	2.89
13	Duke Univ	522	0.6	3.46
14	Univ of British Columbia	512	0.59	3.10
15	Massachusetts Gen Hosp	475	0.55	2.54

Figure 2　Institutions with the most publications and citations related to medical education in 2019 and 2020

3. Authors with the most publications and citations related to medical education in 2019 and 2020（Figure 3）

Ranking	Author	Institution	Number of publications
1	Durning, Steven J.	Uniformed Serv Univ of Hlth Sci	46
2	Sally A. Santen	Virginia Commonwealth Univ	38
3	Ten Cate, Olle	Univ Med Ctr Utrecht	34
4	Park, Yoon Soo	Univ of Illinois	31
5	Cleland, Jennifer	Univ of Aberdeen	29
6	Varpio, Lara	Uniformed Serv Univ of Hlth Sci	26
7	Hauer, Karen E.	Univ of Calif San Francisco	23
8	Roberts, Laura Weiss	Stanford Univ	23
9	Sandhu, Gurjit	Univ of Michigan Hlth Syst	21
10	Balon, Richard	Wayne State Univ	19
11	Dornan, Tim	Queens Univ Belfast	19
12	Eva, Kevin W.	Univ of British Columbia	19
13	Konge, Lars	Univ Copenhagen	19
14	Teunissen, Pim W.	Maastricht Univ	19
15	Ginsburg, Shiphra	Univ of Toronto	18

Ranking	Author	Institution	Number of citations	Average number of citations
1	Rose, Suzanne	Univ of Penn	198	39.60
2	Durning, Steven J.	Uniformed Serv Univ of Hlth Sci	176	3.83
3	Ten Cate, Olle	Univ of Med Ctr Utrecht	168	4.94
4	Bilimoria, Karl Y.	Northwestern Univ	157	9.24
5	Esperto, Francesco	Campus Biomed Univ	151	18.88
6	Ginsburg, Shiphra	Univ of Toronto	146	8.11
7	Yue-Yung Hu	Northwestern Univ	141	11.75
8	Buyske, Jo	Amer Board Surg	135	19.29
9	Hoyt, David B.	Amer Coll Surg	135	22.50
10	Ellis, Ryan J.	Northwestern Univ	130	16.25
11	Hewitt, D. Brock	Northwestern Univ	128	21.33
12	Duma, Narjust	Mayo Clin	127	63.50
13	Varpio, Lara	Uniformed Serv Univ of Hlth Sci	126	4.85
14	Molina, Julian R.	Mayo Clin	126	126.00
15	Santana-Davila	Univ of Washington	126	126.00

Figure 3　Authors with the most publications and citations related to medical education in 2019 and 2020

Note：All authors were considered equally，without distinguishing between first author，corresponding author，or co-author.

4. Highest frequent MeSH terms from publications in medical education in 2019 and 2020（Figure 4）

Ranking	MeSH Term	Frequency	Percentage	Ranking	MeSH Term	Frequency	Percentage
1	Internship and Residency	3986	7.60	21	Pediatrics	355	0.68
2	Students, Medical	2112	4.03	22	Teaching	348	0.66
3	Education, Medical	1983	3.78	23	Psychiatry	347	0.66
4	Education, Medical, Graduate	1650	3.15	24	Surgeons	334	0.64
5	Clinical Competence	1601	3.05	25	Career Choice	331	0.63
6	Education, Medical, Undergraduate	1453	2.77	26	Fellowships and Scholarships	289	0.55
7	Curriculum	1056	2.01	27	Emergency Medicine	277	0.53
8	Physicians	624	1.19	28	Education, Distance	276	0.53
9	Coronavirus Infections	615	1.17	29	Burnout, Professional	272	0.52
10	Pneumonia, Viral	612	1.17	30	Radiology	272	0.52
11	General Surgery	601	1.15	31	Clinical Clerkship	269	0.51
12	Educational Measurement	581	1.11	32	Internal Medicine	250	0.48
13	Simulation Training	502	0.96	33	Anatomy	239	0.46
14	Education, Medical, Continuing	443	0.84	34	Problem-Based Learning	236	0.45
15	Faculty, Medical	426	0.81	35	Physician-Patient Relations	220	0.42
16	Pandemics	426	0.81	36	Biomedical Research	215	0.41
17	Attitude of Health Personnel	417	0.80	37	Betacoronavirus	215	0.41
18	COVID-19	381	0.73	38	Communication	212	0.40
19	Schools, Medical	375	0.72	39	Orthopedics	210	0.40
20	Learning	370	0.71	40	Health Personnel	206	0.39

Figure 4　Highest frequent MeSH terms from publications in medical education in 2019 and 2020

5. Highest frequent MeSH terms clustering of publications in medical education from 2019 and 2020（Figure 5）

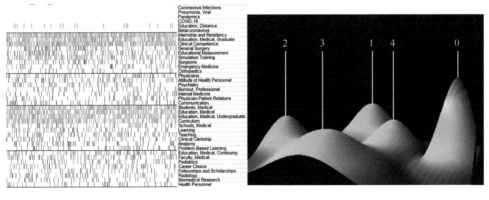

Figure 5　Highest frequent MeSH terms clustering of publications in medical education from 2019 and 2020

Note：The numbers in the right figure indicate the theme categories formed by the highest frequent MeSH terms clustering of publications.

　　Through high frequent MeSH terms clustering，five major themes about international medical education in 2019 and 2020 emerged：

　　（1）The role of distance teaching in medical education under the influence of the COVID-19 pandemic.

　　（2）Application of standardized patients and virtual simulations in the standardized training of residents.

　　（3）Cultivation and evaluation of clinical communication skills of medical staff.

　　（4）Reform of teaching and learning models in human anatomy courses.

　　（5）Others，including career choices and performance-based pay distributions of medical workers.

　　Emerging topic： medical education reform under the COVID-19 pandemic

　　Search Strategy："Education，Medical"[MeSH] OR（*Academic Medicine / Medical Education / Medical Teacher / BMC Medical Education / Journal of Surgical Education / Advances in Health Sciences Education / Teaching and Learning in Medicine / Medical Education Online / Anatomical Sciences Education / Academic Psychiatry*）[Journal] AND "COVID-19"[MeSH].

　　1. Highest frequent MeSH terms from publications in medical education during COVID-19 pandemic in 2019 and 2020（Figure 6）

Ranking	MeSH Term	Frequency	Percentage	Ranking	MeSH Term	Frequency	Percentage
1	Coronavirus Infections	599	8.81	21	Educational Measurement	37	0.54
2	Pneumonia, Viral	596	8.77	22	Dermatology	36	0.53
3	COVID-19	584	8.59	23	Radiology	36	0.53
4	Pandemics	465	6.84	24	Schools, Medical	34	0.50
5	Internship and Residency	422	6.21	25	Ophthalmology	34	0.50
6	Education, Medical	290	4.27	26	Urology	33	0.49
7	Education, Distance	235	3.46	27	Delivery of Health Care	31	0.46
8	Betacoronavirus	211	3.10	28	Anatomy	31	0.46
9	Education, Medical, Graduate	204	3.00	29	Otolaryngology	31	0.46
10	Students, Medical	202	2.97	30	Teaching	30	0.44
11	Education, Medical, Undergraduate	139	2.04	31	Neurosurgery	30	0.44
12	Telemedicine	78	1.15	32	Infection Control	30	0.44
13	Curriculum	68	1.00	33	Physicians	30	0.44
14	Clinical Competence	67	0.99	34	Clinical Clerkship	27	0.40
15	General Surgery	63	0.93	35	Personnel Selection	27	0.40
16	SARS-CoV-2	57	0.84	36	Faculty, Medical	25	0.37
17	Computer-Assisted Instruction	48	0.71	37	Pediatrics	25	0.37
18	Videoconferencing	42	0.62	38	Interviews as Topic	24	0.35
19	Education, Medical, Continuing	39	0.57	39	Surgery, Plastic	22	0.32
20	Fellowships and Scholarships	38	0.56	40	Simulation Training	22	0.32

Figure 6　Highest frequent MeSH terms from publications in medical education during COVID-19 pandemic in 2019 and 2020

2. Top 1% most cited papers in medical education during COVID-19 pandemic in 2019 and 2020（Figure 7）

Ranking	Most cited papers	Frequency
1	Rose S. Medical Student Education in the Time of COVID-19. JAMA. 2020 Jun 2;323(21):2131-2132.	200
2	Chick R C, Clifton G T, Peace K M, Propper B W, Hale D F, Alseidi A A, Vreeland T J. Using Technology to Maintain the Education of Residents During the COVID-19 Pandemic. J Surg Educ. 2020 Jul-Aug;77(4):729-732.	117
3	Fix O K, Hameed B, Fontana R J, Kwok R M, McGuire B M, Mulligan D C, Pratt D S, Russo M W, Schilsky M L, Verna E C, Loomba R, Cohen D E, Bezerra J A, Reddy K R, Chung R T. Clinical Best Practice Advice for Hepatology and Liver Transplant Providers During the COVID-19 Pandemic: AASLD Expert Panel Consensus Statement. Hepatology. 2020 Jul;72(1):287-304.	89
4	Ahmed H, Allaf M, Elghazaly H. COVID-19 and medical education. Lancet Infect Dis. 2020 Jul; 20(7): 777-778.	80
5	Almarzooq Z I, Lopes M, Kochar A. Virtual Learning During the COVID-19 Pandemic: A Disruptive Technology in Graduate Medical Education. J Am Coll Cardiol. 2020 May 26;75(20):2635-2638.	60
6	Porpiglia F, Checcucci E, Amparore D, Verri P, Campi R, Claps F, Esperto F, Fiori C, Carrieri G, Ficarra V, Mario Scarpa R, Dasgupta P. Slowdown of urology residents' learning curve during the COVID-19 emergency. BJU Int. 2020 Jun;125(6):e15-e17.	52
7	Amparore D, Claps F, Cacciamani G E, Esperto F, Fiori C, Liguori G, Serni S, Trombetta C, Carini M, Porpiglia F, Checcucci E, Campi R. Impact of the COVID-19 pandemic on urology residency training in Italy. Minerva Urol Nefrol. 2020 Aug;72(4):505-509.	52
8	Kogan M, Klein S E, Hannon C P, Nolte M T. Orthopaedic Education During the COVID-19 Pandemic. J Am Acad Orthop Surg. 2020 Jun 1;28(11):e456-e464.	50
9	Evans D J R, Bay B H, Wilson T D, Smith C F, Lachman N, Pawlina W. Going Virtual to Support Anatomy Education: A STOPGAP in the Midst of the COVID-19 Pandemic. Anat Sci Educ. 2020 May;13(3):279-283.	49
10	Nassar A H, Zern N K, McIntyre L K, Lynge D, Smith C A, Petersen R P, Horvath K D, Wood D E. Emergency Restructuring of a General Surgery Residency Program During the Coronavirus Disease 2019 Pandemic: The University of Washington Experience. JAMA Surg. 2020 Jul 1;155(7):624-627.	48
11	Alvin M D, George E, Deng F, Warhadpande S, Lee S I. The Impact of COVID-19 on Radiology Trainees. Radiology. 2020 Aug;296(2):246-248.	48
12	Pather N, Blyth P, Chapman J A, Dayal M R, Flack N A M S, Fogg Q A, Green R A, Hulme A K, Johnson I P, Meyer A J, Morley J W, Shortland P J, Štrkalj G, Štrkalj M, Valter K, Webb A L, Woodley S J, Lazarus M D. Forced Disruption of Anatomy Education in Australia and New Zealand: An Acute Response to the COVID-19 Pandemic. Anat Sci Educ. 2020 May; 13(3): 284-300.	47
13	Dedeilia A, Sotiropoulos M G, Hanrahan J G, Janga D, Dedeilias P, Sideris M. Medical and Surgical Education Challenges and Innovations in the COVID-19 Era: A Systematic Review. In Vivo. 2020 Jun; 34(3 Suppl):1603-1611.	45
14	Ripp J, Peccoralo L, Charney D. Attending to the Emotional Well-Being of the Health Care Workforce in a New York City Health System During the COVID-19 Pandemic. Acad Med. 2020 Aug; 95(8): 1136-1139.	41

Figure 7 Top 1% most cited papers in medical education during COVID-19 pandemic in
2019 and 2020

3. Highest frequent MeSH terms clustering of publications in medical education during COVID-19 pandemic in 2019 and 2020（Figure 8）

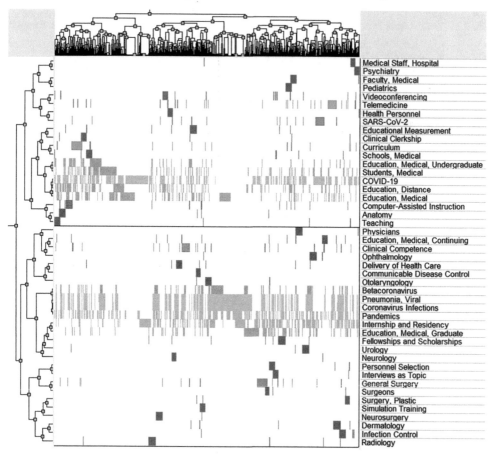

Figure 8　High frequent MeSH terms clustering of publications in medical education during
COVID-19 pandemic in 2019 and 2020

Through high frequent MeSH terms clustering, two major themes about international medical education during COVID-19 pandemic in 2019 and 2020 emerged：

（1）Impact of COVID-19 pandemic on undergraduate medical education.

（2）Impact of the COVID-19 pandemic on clinical practice（graduated and continuing medical education）.

Analysis of medical education challenges during the COVID-19 pandemic

The COVID-19 pandemic is a "great test" and "severe test" to the sufficiency and supporting ability of China's medical education, revealing many challenges that China's medical education is facing at present. However, from the dialectical perspective of "danger" and "opportunity", it can be regarded as a favorable opportunity to force the reform and development of medical education.

（1）The distribution of physician resources remains uneven

The COVID-19 epidemic has highlighted the uncoordinated characteristics of physician resources in China, with significant differences in development levels among provinces, regions, and cities, as well as between urban and rural areas. There is also a lack of top-notch innovative medical professionals. First, there are regional disparities in physician supply and demand. The numbers of doctors in eastern regions such as Beijing, Zhejiang, and Shanghai are relatively sufficient, while there is a shortage in central and western provinces such as Yunnan, Guangxi, and Gansu. Second, there is blatant "polarization" of physician groups. In other words, the number of doctors per 1,000 people in rural areas is only 45 percent of that in urban areas, and the number of doctors per 1,000 people in urban areas is also insufficient. Third, influenced by the traditional planned enrollment system, clinical medicine programs lack the training ability of top high-level innovative talents. In China, the enrollment scale of the eight-year clinical medicine doctoral program is small, and there are not enough qualified universities to admit students. At present, only 14 universities can enroll students for the eight-year program, and the actual enrollment in each university is relatively low in proportion to overall medical enrollment.

（2）There are "hidden dangers" in the development environment of medical and health care services

The COVID-19 outbreak reflects environmental problems that hinder the development of health care, such as low government financial investment and lack of respect for doctors. Firstly, financial investment in health care needs to be increased. Compared with developed countries such as the United States and Japan, China's medical and health expenditure accounts for a small proportion of the total government expenditure, and the proportion of total health expenditure to GDP is small and relatively regressive. Secondly, there is insufficient government investment in university training programs, and there is a large gap between the funds of affiliated universities versus local universities. Thirdly, there is an urgent need to improve and reform the social status of doctors and the social ethos of respecting and valuing medical treatment. The loss of equality between doctors and patients and the gradual decline of social status for doctors have greatly weakened the appeal, cultivation, and transference of medical education, especially for clinicians.

（3）Planning and construction of the public health system lack sufficient attention

The COVID-19 pandemic has exposed the challenges in China's public health management system. The small scale and insufficient strength of the disease prevention and control institutions, especially the lack of professional staff and the pressure of the brain drain, have become the main bottlenecks restricting the role of the public health system in epidemic prevention and control. First, the management system and mechanism of public health undertakings are constrained, which squeeze and weaken to a certain extent the development space and key discourse power of professional institutions. Second, the number of disease prevention and control institutions in China and the reservoir of staff showed a decreasing trend, resulting in a large number of "surprise" recruitments during the epidemic. Third, there is a worrying emigration of public-health doctors. Low salary and loss of sense of professional belonging have become the main reasons for the lack of willingness for participation and ability to stay engaged in highly educated graduates and public health practitioners.

（4）There are weak links in the training process of medical professionals

The harrowing casualties in the COVID-19 pandemic have revealed the inadequacy and incompleteness of the medical training system for "big health" and "full life cycle". Gaps in the basic public health knowledge of clinical medical personnel and the prevention and control skills of emerging infectious diseases need to be addressed urgently. First, in the process of training clinical medical professionals, the general knowledge structure tends to lean towards treatment rather than prevention, and shortcomings in technology limit the practical abilities of protective health. Secondly, there is an obvious disconnection between treatment and prevention in the professional training of public health and preventive medicine personnel, especially seen in the weak application of epidemic prevention and disease resistance.

In the future, comprehensively enhancing and diversifying the supply capacity of clinicians, taking multiple measures to improve the quality of medical education, reconstructing the security and credibility of the public health system, and optimizing the external governance mechanism of medical education have become the main approaches to deepen the reform and accelerate the innovative development of medical education.

II. Research fronts of doctor's common competency

Medical knowledge and life-long learning

Search Strategy：（Knowledge [MeSH] OR Learning [MeSH]）AND（Physicians

[MeSH] OR Internship and Residency [MeSH] OR Students，Medical [MeSH]）.

Time Range: 2011-01-01–2020-12-31.

1. Highest frequent MeSH terms from publications about medical knowledge and life-long learning between 2011 and 2020（Figure 9）

Ranking	MeSH Term	Frequency	Percentage	Ranking	MeSH Term	Frequency	Percentage
1	Students, Medical	2206	8.80	21	Computer-Assisted Instruction	179	0.71
2	Learning	1219	4.86	22	Clinical Clerkship	176	0.70
3	Internship and Residency	1155	4.61	23	Formative Feedback	176	0.70
4	Education, Medical, Undergraduate	1148	4.58	24	Schools, Medical	137	0.55
				25	Education, Medical, Continuing	134	0.53
5	Clinical Competence	1064	4.24	26	Communication	128	0.51
6	Problem-Based Learning	772	3.08	27	Physician-Patient Relations	128	0.51
7	Education, Medical	602	2.40	28	Pediatrics	128	0.51
8	Teaching	566	2.26	29	Interprofessional Relations	126	0.50
9	Education, Medical, Graduate	481	1.92	30	Computer Simulation	112	0.45
10	Educational Measurement	432	1.72	31	General Practitioners	110	0.44
11	Curriculum	430	1.71	32	Peer Group	106	0.42
12	Physicians	423	1.69	33	Knowledge	99	0.39
13	Learning Curve	295	1.18	34	Internal Medicine	98	0.39
14	Surgeons	247	0.98	35	Problem Solving	94	0.37
15	Attitude of Health Personnel	236	0.94	36	Emergency Medicine	92	0.37
16	General Surgery	211	0.84	37	Internet	90	0.36
17	Anatomy	198	0.79	38	Health Knowledge, Attitudes, Practice	89	0.35
18	Faculty, Medical	196	0.78				
19	Laparoscopy	189	0.75	39	Robotic Surgical Procedures	89	0.35
20	Simulation Training	184	0.73	40	Anesthesiology	87	0.35

Figure 9　Highest frequent MeSH terms from publications about medical knowledge and life-long learning between 2011 and 2020

2. Highest frequent MeSH terms clustering of publications about medical knowledge and life-long learning between 2011 and 2020（Figure 10）

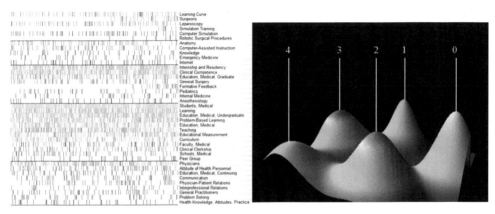

Figure 10　Highest frequent MeSH terms clustering of publications about medical knowledge and life-long learning between 2011 and 2020

Through highest frequent MeSH terms clustering，five major themes in medical knowledge and life-long learning emerged：

（1）Impact of robot-assisted surgery on the learning curve of surgeons.

（2）Application of web（online）teaching resources in the teaching of human anatomy.

（3）Effect of clinical skills training for residents.

（4）Application and impact evaluation of teaching methods such as PBL and peer learning in medical education.

（5）Others，including interprofessional education and solutions to professional dilemmas.

Clinical skills and patient care

Search Strategy：（Clinical Competence [Majr：NoExp] OR Patient Care [Majr：NoExp]）AND（Physicians [MeSH] OR Internship and Residency [MeSH] OR Students，Medical [MeSH]）.

Time Range: 2011-01-01–2020-12-31.

1. Highest frequent MeSH terms from publications about clinical skills and patient care between 2011 and 2020（Figure 11）

Ranking	MeSH Term	Frequency	Percentage	Ranking	MeSH Term	Frequency	Percentage
1	Clinical Competence	8501	19.32	21	General Practitioners	236	0.54
2	Internship and Residency	3202	7.28	22	Education, Medical, Continuing	226	0.51
3	Students, Medical	1412	3.21	23	Communication	222	0.50
4	Physicians	1233	2.80	24	Physician-Patient Relations	215	0.49
5	Education, Medical, Graduate	1187	2.70	25	Teaching	206	0.47
6	Educational Measurement	878	2.00	26	Clinical Clerkship	203	0.46
7	Education, Medical, Undergraduate	719	1.63	27	Anesthesiology	194	0.44
8	General Surgery	645	1.47	28	Competency-Based Education	193	0.44
9	Curriculum	542	1.23	29	Practice Patterns, Physicians'	184	0.42
10	Attitude of Health Personnel	510	1.16	30	Faculty, Medical	182	0.41
11	Surgeons	502	1.14	31	Family Practice	178	0.40
12	Patient Care	419	0.95	32	Orthopedics	174	0.40
13	Education, Medical	359	0.82	33	Learning	173	0.39
14	Simulation Training	357	0.81	34	Ophthalmology	172	0.39
15	Laparoscopy	357	0.81	35	Radiology	149	0.34
16	Pediatrics	311	0.71	36	Surveys and Questionnaires	140	0.32
17	Internal Medicine	298	0.68	37	Physicians, Primary Care	140	0.32
18	Emergency Medicine	262	0.60	38	Certification	133	0.30
19	Computer Simulation	256	0.58	39	Patient Simulation	127	0.29
20	Health Knowledge, Attitudes, Practice	238	0.54	40	Learning Curve	123	0.28

Figure 11　Highest frequent MeSH terms from publications about clinical skills and patient care between 2011 and 2020

2. Highest frequent MeSH terms clustering of publications about clinical skills and patient care between 2011 and 2020（Figure 12）

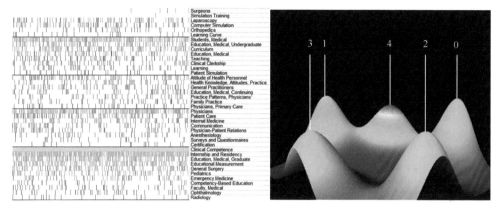

Figure 12　Highest frequent MeSH terms clustering of publications about clinical skills and patient care between 2011 and 2020

Through highest frequent MeSH terms clustering, five major themes in clinical skills and patient care have emerged in the recent ten years:

（1）Development and application of clinical skills training and assessment tools.

（2）Application of standardized patients in the teaching and evaluation of medical students during clinical clerkship.

（3）Medical knowledge and clinical skills training for healthcare workers.

（4）Investigation on the influencing factors of health care quality and physician-patient relations.

（5）Training and evaluation of clinical skills in residents and medical residents.

Disease prevention and health promotion

Search Strategy：Preventive Health Services [MeSH] AND（Physicians [MeSH] OR Internship and Residency [MeSH] OR Students，Medical [MeSH]）.

Time Range: 2011-01-01–2020-12-31.

1. Highest frequent MeSH terms from publications about disease prevention and health promotion between 2011 and 2020（Figure 13）

Ranking	MeSH Term	Frequency	Percentage	Ranking	MeSH Term	Frequency	Percentage
1	Physicians	671	3.79	21	Early Detection of Cancer	114	0.64
2	Attitude of Health Personnel	466	2.63	22	Communication	102	0.58
3	Health Knowledge, Attitudes, Practice	454	2.56	23	Breast Neoplasms	99	0.56
				24	Influenza, Human	99	0.56
4	Mass Screening	412	2.33	25	Neoplasms	94	0.53
5	Students, Medical	378	2.14	26	Preventive Health Services	93	0.53
6	Health Promotion	375	2.12	27	Influenza Vaccines	90	0.51
7	Patient Education as Topic	365	2.06	28	Pediatricians	85	0.48
8	General Practitioners	365	2.06	29	Smoking Cessation	85	0.48
9	Practice Patterns, Physicians'	357	2.02	30	Health Literacy	83	0.47
10	Vaccination	305	1.72	31	Referral and Consultation	82	0.46
11	Physicians, Primary Care	286	1.62	32	Health Personnel	81	0.46
12	Primary Health Care	272	1.54	33	Patient Acceptance of Health Care	79	0.45
13	Internship and Residency	252	1.42				
14	Physician-Patient Relations	185	1.04	34	Papillomavirus Vaccines	79	0.45
15	Clinical Competence	148	0.84	35	Pediatrics	78	0.44
16	Genetic Testing	137	0.77	36	Counseling	77	0.43
17	Health Education	134	0.76	37	Parents	76	0.43
18	Physicians, Family	122	0.69	38	Surgeons	72	0.41
19	Physician's Role	121	0.68	39	Guideline Adherence	70	0.40
20	HIV Infections	117	0.66	40	Internet	70	0.40

Figure 13   Highest frequent MeSH terms from publications about disease prevention and health promotion between 2011 and 2020

2. Highest frequent MeSH terms clustering of publications about disease prevention and health promotion between 2011 and 2020（Figure 14）

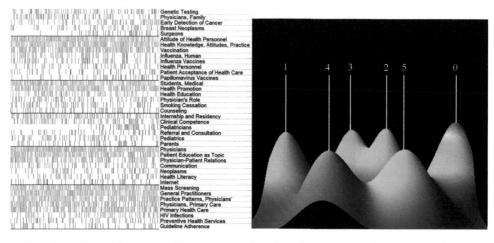

Figure 14   Highest frequent MeSH terms clustering of publications about disease prevention and health promotion between 2011 and 2020

Through highest frequent MeSH terms clustering, six major themes in disease prevention and health promotion have emerged in the recent ten years:

（1）Implementing early cancer screening and developing guidelines for cancer prevention and treatment.

（2）A survey on the acceptance of influenza vaccination among primary healthcare workers.

（3）Health education and smoking cessation activities for physicians and medical students.

（4）Internet-based health literacy and patient education.

（5）Campaigns for screening and prevention of AIDS.

（6）Others, including training in vaccine safety and promotion of free vaccination programs.

Information and management

Search Strategy:（Information Management [MeSH] OR Self-Management [MeSH] OR Time Management [MeSH] OR Leadership [MeSH]）AND（Physicians [MeSH] OR Internship and Residency [MeSH] OR Students, Medical [MeSH]）.

Time Range: 2011-01-01–2020-12-31.

1. Highest frequent MeSH terms from publications about information and management between 2011 and 2020（Figure 15）

Ranking	MeSH Term	Frequency	Percentage	Ranking	MeSH Term	Frequency	Percentage
1	Physicians	1438	5.52	21	Data Collection	180	0.69
2	Internship and Residency	1066	4.09	22	General Surgery	169	0.65
3	Leadership	864	3.32	23	Communication	162	0.62
4	Students, Medical	810	3.11	24	Curriculum	157	0.60
5	Attitude of Health Personnel	800	3.07	25	Narration	150	0.58
6	General Practitioners	447	1.72	26	Decision-Making	143	0.55
7	Clinical Competence	411	1.58	27	Interprofessional Relations	142	0.55
8	Physicians, Women	294	1.13	28	Personnel Selection	139	0.53
9	Physician-Patient Relations	279	1.07	29	Family Practice	134	0.51
10	Education, Medical, Graduate	277	1.06	30	Physicians, Family	133	0.51
11	Faculty, Medical	255	0.98	31	Pediatrics	130	0.50
12	Health Knowledge, Attitudes, Practice	250	0.96	32	Delivery of Health Care	130	0.50
13	Education, Medical, Undergraduate	245	0.94	33	Patient Care Team	120	0.46
14	Practice Patterns, Physicians'	230	0.88	34	Learning	114	0.44
15	Primary Health Care	227	0.87	35	Teaching	113	0.43
16	Interviews as Topic	226	0.87	36	Schools, Medical	112	0.43
17	Education, Medical	213	0.82	37	Internal Medicine	111	0.43
18	Surgeons	210	0.81	38	Physician's Role	111	0.43
19	Career Choice	196	0.75	39	Educational Measurement	104	0.40
20	Physicians, Primary Care	188	0.72	40	Neoplasms	103	0.40

Figure 15　Highest frequent MeSH terms from publications about information and management between 2011 and 2020

2. Highest frequent MeSH terms clustering of publications about information and management between 2011 and 2020（Figure 16）

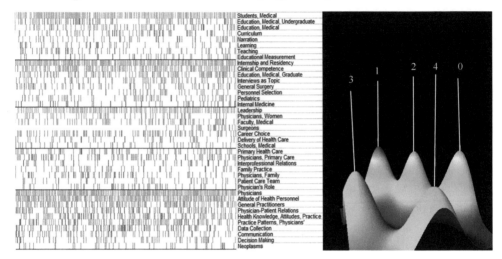

Figure 16　Highest frequent MeSH terms clustering of publications about information and management between 2011 and 2020

Through Highest frequent MeSH terms clustering, five major themes in information and management have emerged in the recent ten years:

（1）The application of narrative medicine in medical education.

（2）Factors influencing admission and recruitment of residents.

（3）The relationship between gender and leadership.

（4）The role of the family doctors in primary health care.

（5）Research on how physicians make clinical decisions in clinical diagnosis and treatment.

Interpersonal communication

Search Strategy: Communication [MeSH] AND Interpersonal Relations [MeSH] AND（Physicians [MeSH] OR Internship and Residency [MeSH] OR Students, Medical [MeSH]）.

Time Range: 2011-01-01–2020-12-31.

1. Highest frequent MeSH terms from publications about interpersonal communication between 2011 and 2020（Figure 17）

Ranking	MeSH Term	Frequency	Percentage	Ranking	MeSH Term	Frequency	Percentage
1	Physician-Patient Relations	1222	6.16	21	Referral and Consultation	134	0.68
2	Communication	1164	5.87	22	Patient Satisfaction	126	0.64
3	Physicians	1120	5.65	23	Patient-Centered Care	125	0.63
4	Students, Medical	466	2.35	24	Conflict of Interest	120	0.61
5	Attitude of Health Personnel	463	2.34	25	Education, Medical	119	0.60
6	Internship and Residency	422	2.13	26	Truth Disclosure	105	0.53
7	Interdisciplinary Communication	392	1.98	27	Practice Patterns, Physicians'	103	0.52
8	Clinical Competence	314	1.58	28	Empathy	103	0.52
9	Disclosure	302	1.52	29	Oncologists	100	0.50
10	Interprofessional Relations	276	1.39	30	Terminal Care	97	0.49
11	General Practitioners	274	1.38	31	Drug Industry	96	0.48
12	Neoplasms	211	1.06	32	Education, Medical, Graduate	96	0.48
13	Patient Care Team	202	1.02	33	Professional-Family Relations	94	0.47
14	Education, Medical, Undergraduate	173	0.87	34	Curriculum	92	0.46
15	Health Knowledge, Attitudes, Practice	164	0.83	35	Communication Barriers	87	0.44
16	Physicians, Primary Care	159	0.80	36	Pediatrics	87	0.44
17	Primary Health Care	154	0.78	37	Physician's Role	84	0.42
18	Decision-Making	146	0.74	38	Patient Participation	84	0.42
19	Surgeons	143	0.72	39	General Surgery	80	0.40
20	Cooperative Behavior	138	0.70	40	Negotiating	80	0.40

Figure 17　Highest frequent MeSH terms from publications about interpersonal communication between 2011 and 2020

2. Highest frequent MeSH terms clustering of publications about interpersonal communication between 2011 and 2020（Figure 18）

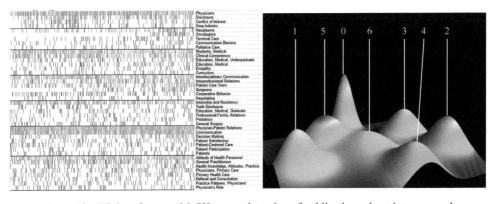

Figure 18　Highest frequent MeSH terms clustering of publications about interpersonal communication between 2011 and 2020

Through highest frequent MeSH terms clustering, seven major themes in interpersonal communication emerged:

(1) Physician Payments Sunshine Act—an important measure to reveal conflicts of interest between health care providers and the pharmaceutical industry.

(2) Barriers in communication between health care workers and cancer patients regarding end-of-life care.

(3) Impact of hidden curriculum on clinical skills (e.g., patient interactions) and empathy in medical students.

(4) Interprofessional communication and cooperation in physicians.

(5) Communication between physicians and patients' families and the development and application of related communication skills assessment tools.

(6) The relationship between physician communication styles and quality of patient participation in clinical decision-making.

(7) The role of health care providers in patient health management.

Teamwork

Search Strategy: (Cooperative Behavior [MeSH] OR Patient Care Team [MeSH] OR Intersectoral Collaboration[MeSH] OR Interprofessional Relations[MeSH]) AND (Physicians [MeSH] OR Internship and Residency [MeSH] OR Students, Medical [MeSH]).
Time Range: 2011-01-01–2020-12-31.

1. Highest frequent MeSH terms from publications about team work between 2011 and 2020 (Figure 19)

Ranking	MeSH Term	Frequency	Percentage	Ranking	MeSH Term	Frequency	Percentage
1	Interprofessional Relations	1165	4.79	21	Referral and Consultation	136	0.56
2	Physicians	1093	4.50	22	Patient-Centered Care	131	0.54
3	Patient Care Team	943	3.88	23	Pediatrics	124	0.51
4	Internship and Residency	730	3.00	24	Hospitalists	123	0.51
5	Attitude of Health Personnel	636	2.62	25	Practice Patterns, Physicians'	121	0.50
6	Students, Medical	635	2.61	26	Quality Improvement	119	0.49
7	Cooperative Behavior	614	2.53	27	Physician's Role	118	0.49
8	Interdisciplinary Communication	392	1.61	28	Physician-Patient Relations	116	0.48
9	Clinical Competence	355	1.46	29	Delivery of Health Care	116	0.48
10	Primary Health Care	332	1.37	30	Nurses	110	0.45
11	General Practitioners	317	1.30	31	Faculty, Medical	110	0.45
12	Pharmacists	263	1.08	32	Family Practice	110	0.45
13	Education, Medical	230	0.95	33	Patient Safety	110	0.45
14	Communication	217	0.89	34	Leadership	107	0.44
15	Education, Medical, Undergraduate	213	0.88	35	Learning	98	0.40
				36	Drug Industry	97	0.40
16	Surgeons	208	0.86	37	Psychiatry	97	0.40
17	Physicians, Primary Care	198	0.81	38	Health Personnel	97	0.40
18	Education, Medical, Graduate	193	0.79	39	Health Knowledge, Attitudes, Practice	97	0.40
19	General Surgery	160	0.66				
20	Curriculum	143	0.59	40	Students, Nursing	96	0.39

Figure 19　Highest frequent MeSH terms from publications about team work between 2011 and 2020

2. Highest frequent MeSH terms clustering of publications about teamwork between 2011 and 2020（Figure 20）

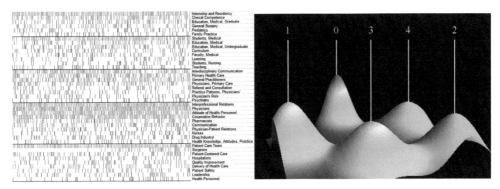

Figure 20　Highest frequent MeSH terms clustering of publications about team work between 2011 and 2020

Through highest frequent MeSH terms clustering, five major themes in teamwork have emerged in the recent ten years:

（1）Methods of strengthening clinical skills training for primary healthcare workers.

（2）Curriculum development and application of interprofessional collaboration between medical students and nursing students.

（3）Interprofessional communication and collaboration between clinicians and primary healthcare workers.

（4）Attitudes of clinicians, nurses, and pharmacists toward interprofessional collaboration.

（5）Challenges and opportunities for leadership in patient care teams.

Research

Search Strategy：Research [MeSH] AND（Physicians [MeSH] OR Internship and Residency [MeSH] OR Students, Medical [MeSH]）.

Time Range: 2011-01-01–2020-12-31.

1. Highest frequent MeSH terms from publications about research between 2011 and 2020（Figure 21）

Ranking	MeSH Term	Frequency	Percentage	Ranking	MeSH Term	Frequency	Percentage
1	Physicians	1500	4.56	21	Faculty, Medical	205	0.62
2	Attitude of Health Personnel	1108	3.37	22	Curriculum	200	0.61
3	Biomedical Research	1099	3.34	23	General Surgery	190	0.58
4	Students, Medical	1081	3.29	24	Research Personnel	185	0.56
5	Internship and Residency	1019	3.10	25	Decision-Making	183	0.56
6	General Practitioners	758	2.30	26	Neoplasms	180	0.55
7	Primary Health Care	493	1.50	27	Physicians, Family	179	0.54
8	Clinical Competence	445	1.35	28	Pediatrics	174	0.53
9	Education, Medical, Undergraduate	385	1.17	29	General Practice	170	0.52
10	Physician-Patient Relations	348	1.06	30	Interprofessional Relations	161	0.49
11	Practice Patterns, Physicians'	322	0.98	31	Learning	153	0.47
12	Education, Medical, Graduate	318	0.97	32	Family Practice	151	0.46
13	Surgeons	302	0.92	33	Research Design	148	0.45
14	Research	278	0.84	34	Qualitative Research	125	0.38
15	Health Knowledge, Attitudes, Practice	268	0.81	35	Nurses	125	0.38
				36	Palliative Care	125	0.38
16	Outcome Assessment, Health Care	260	0.79	37	Referral and Consultation	122	0.37
17	Physicians, Primary Care	257	0.78				
18	Education, Medical	255	0.78	38	Internal Medicine	120	0.36
19	Career Choice	222	0.67	39	Quality of Health Care	119	0.36
20	Communication	213	0.65	40	Schools, Medical	117	0.36

Figure 21　Highest frequent MeSH terms from publications about research between 2011 and 2020

2. Highest frequent MeSH terms clustering of publications about research between 2011 and 2020（Figure 22）

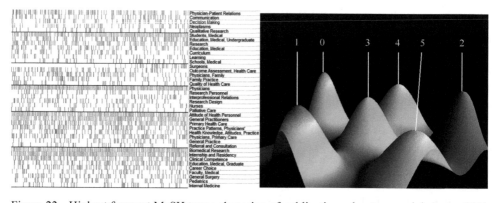

Figure 22　Highest frequent MeSH terms clustering of publications about research between 2011 and 2020

Through highest frequent MeSH terms clustering, six major themes in research have emerged in the recent ten years:

（1）Communication and decision-making between physicians and critically-ill patients on the issue of informing patients.

（2）Impact of explicit curriculum and hidden curriculum on medical students' learning goals and learning outcomes.

（3）Effectiveness of family physicians on health care quality and outcomes for patients.

（4）Health care workers' perceptions and understandings of palliative care.

（5）Experience of general practitioners in the treatment of mental health problems in children and adolescents.

（6）Impact of practice environment on academic performance and career choice of residents.

Core values and professionalism

Search Strategy：（Value of Life [MeSH] OR Social Values [MeSH] OR Codes of Ethics [MeSH] AND Ethics, Professional [MeSH] OR Humanism [MeSH] OR Professional Misconduct [MeSH] OR Altruism [MeSH] OR Professionalism[tiab] OR "professional performance*" [tiab] OR "professional behavior*" [tiab] OR "unprofessional behavior*" OR "professional attitude*" [tiab] OR "professional identity formation" [tiab]）AND（Physicians [MeSH] OR Internship and Residency [MeSH] OR Students, Medical [MeSH]）.

Time Range: 2011-01-01–2020-12-31.

1. Highest frequent MeSH terms from publications about core values and professionalism between 2011 and 2020（Figure 23）

Ranking	MeSH Term	Frequency	Percentage	Ranking	MeSH Term	Frequency	Percentage
1	Students, Medical	751	6.65	21	Altruism	79	0.70
2	Physicians	679	6.01	22	Social Media	79	0.70
3	Internship and Residency	672	5.95	23	Physician's Role	78	0.69
4	Clinical Competence	387	3.43	24	Clinical Clerkship	72	0.64
5	Professionalism	287	2.54	25	Teaching	68	0.60
6	General Surgery	287	2.54	26	Interprofessional Relations	63	0.56
7	Professional Misconduct	272	2.41	27	Communication	61	0.54
8	Education, Medical, Undergraduate	268	2.37	28	Career Choice	59	0.52
				29	Empathy	59	0.52
9	Attitude of Health Personnel	219	1.94	30	Burnout, Professional	56	0.50
10	Education, Medical, Graduate	212	1.88	31	Health Knowledge, Attitudes, Practice	54	0.48
11	Physician-Patient Relations	196	1.74				
12	Education, Medical	184	1.63	32	Orthopedics	52	0.46
13	Curriculum	153	1.35	33	Social Identification	50	0.44
14	Ethics, Medical	149	1.32	34	Pediatrics	50	0.44
15	Professional Competence	138	1.22	35	Practice Patterns, Physicians'	47	0.42
16	Educational Measurement	119	1.05	36	Scientific Misconduct	44	0.39
17	Faculty, Medical	112	0.99	37	Learning	43	0.38
18	Humanism	101	0.89	38	Surveys and Questionnaires	43	0.38
19	Surgeons	88	0.78	39	Delivery of Health Care	42	0.37
20	Schools, Medical	84	0.74	40	General Practitioners	42	0.37

Figure 23　Highest frequent MeSH terms from publications about core values and professionalism between 2011 and 2020

2. Highest frequent MeSH terms clustering of publications about core values and professionalism between 2011 and 2020（Figure 24）

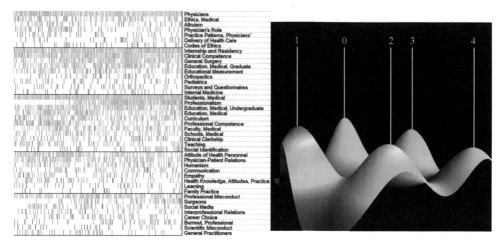

Figure 24　Highest frequent MeSH terms clustering of publications about core values and professionalism between 2011 and 2020

Through highest frequent MeSH terms clustering, five major themes in core values and professionalism have emerged in the recent ten years：

（1）The physician's role and ethical attributes of professionalism.

（2）Development and application of professionalism survey tools for residents.

（3）Professionalism and its training models within different cultural contexts.

（4）Professionalism in medical education research and practice（e.g., humanitarianism, empathy）.

（5）Professional misconduct（including academic misconduct）and the status and coping strategies of burnout in physicians.

Ⅲ. Special topic：global research on medical educational technology

Methods

1. Search Strategy

Search Strategy："Education, Medical" [MeSH] OR（*Academic Medicine / Medical Education / Medical Teacher / BMC Medical Education / Journal of Surgical Education / Advances in Health Sciences Education / Teaching and Learning in Medicine / Medical Education Online / Anatomical Sciences Education / Academic*

Psychiatry）[Journal] AND "Educational Technology" [MeSH].

2. Time Range

2011-01-01–2020-12-31.

3. Statistical Method

CiteSpace was used to analyze bibliometric data, such as number of publications per country/region, per institution, and per author. High frequency MeSH terms clustering was conducted on the main MeSH terms included in literature from the last decade（2011–2020）. Co-citation clustering was performed on the top most cited papers from the last decade（2011–2020）.

Scope of literature and research fronts

1. Countries with the most publications in medical educational technology in the recent ten years（2011–2020）（Figure 25）

Ranking	Country/Region	Number of publications	Betweenness centrality
1	USA	721	0.69
2	Canada	183	0.38
3	England	138	0.36
4	Germany	73	0.05
5	Netherlands	62	0.15
6	Australia	60	0.07
7	PRC	49	0.04
8	Switzerland	34	0.05
9	Japan	32	0.00
10	France	31	0.02
11	Brazil	30	0.01
12	Republic of Korea	27	0.03
13	Spain	23	0.02
14	Italy	21	0.03
15	India	21	0.00

Figure 25   Countries with the most publications in medical educational technology in the recent ten years（2011–2020）

Note：CiteSpace nodes（left）represent countries/regions（publications per time slice, with size of node reflecting cumulative number of publications）. Each ring represents a single time slice（1 year）, from blue（2010）to red（2019）. Thickness of time slice ring is proportional to the number of publications in that particular time slice（1 year）. Links between different countries/regions represent cooperative relationships. Betweenness centrality（right）captures how much a given node is in between others. Greater value of betweenness centrality meant greater importance the node has in the network and direct closer cooperation with other nodes.

2. Institutions with the most publications in medical educational technology in the recent ten years（2011–2020）（Figure 26）

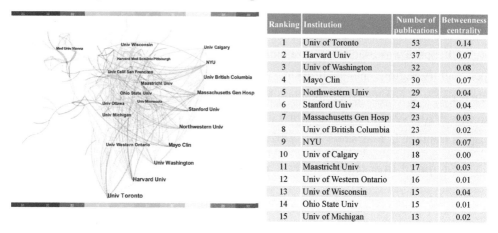

Ranking	Institution	Number of publications	Betweenness centrality
1	Univ of Toronto	53	0.14
2	Harvard Univ	37	0.07
3	Univ of Washington	32	0.08
4	Mayo Clin	30	0.07
5	Northwestern Univ	29	0.04
6	Stanford Univ	24	0.04
7	Massachusetts Gen Hosp	23	0.03
8	Univ of British Columbia	23	0.02
9	NYU	19	0.07
10	Univ of Calgary	18	0.00
11	Maastricht Univ	17	0.03
12	Univ of Western Ontario	16	0.01
13	Univ of Wisconsin	15	0.04
14	Ohio State Univ	15	0.01
15	Univ of Michigan	13	0.02

Figure 26　Institutions with the most publications in medical educational technology in the recent ten years（2011–2020）

Note：CiteSpace visualization on the left shows the distribution of institutions with the most publications（per time slice of 1 year）and close cooperation between different institutions.

3. Authors with the most publications in medical educational technology in the recent ten years（2011–2020）（Figure 27）

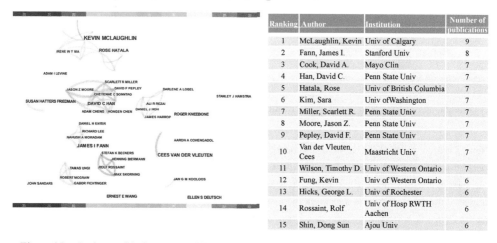

Ranking	Author	Institution	Number of publications
1	McLaughlin, Kevin	Univ of Calgary	9
2	Fann, James I.	Stanford Univ	8
3	Cook, David A.	Mayo Clin	7
4	Han, David C.	Penn State Univ	7
5	Hatala, Rose	Univ of British Columbia	7
6	Kim, Sara	Univ ofWashington	7
7	Miller, Scarlett R.	Penn State Univ	7
8	Moore, Jason Z.	Penn State Univ	7
9	Pepley, David F.	Penn State Univ	7
10	Van der Vleuten, Cees	Maastricht Univ	7
11	Wilson, Timothy D.	Univ of Western Ontario	7
12	Fung, Kevin	Univ of Western Ontario	6
13	Hicks, George L.	Univ of Rochester	6
14	Rossaint, Rolf	Univ of Hosp RWTH Aachen	6
15	Shin, Dong Sun	Ajou Univ	6

Figure 27　Authors with the most publications in medical educational technology in the recent ten years（2011–2020）

Note：CiteSpace visualization on the left shows the distribution of authors with the most publications（per time slice of 1 year）and close cooperation between different authors.

4. Highest frequent MeSH terms from publications in medical educational technology in the recent ten years（2011–2020）（Figure 28）

Ranking	MeSH Term	Frequency	Percentage	Ranking	MeSH Term	Frequency	Percentage
1	Clinical Competence	408	4.87	21	Anesthesiology	79	0.94
2	Internship and Residency	368	4.39	22	Patient Simulation	79	0.94
3	Models, Anatomic	350	4.17	23	Curriculum	79	0.94
4	Education, Medical	328	3.91	24	Learning	68	0.81
5	Education, Medical, Undergraduate	258	3.08	25	Audiovisual Aids	67	0.80
				26	Motion Pictures	65	0.78
6	Education, Medical, Graduate	257	3.07	27	Cardiopulmonary Resuscitation	61	0.73
7	Manikins	196	2.34				
8	Students, Medical	195	2.33	28	Emergency Medicine	57	0.68
9	Simulation Training	184	2.19	29	Intubation, Intratracheal	56	0.67
10	Teaching	165	1.97	30	Laparoscopy	56	0.67
11	Computer Simulation	147	1.75	31	Imaging, Three-Dimensional	52	0.62
12	Computer-Assisted Instruction	114	1.36	32	Psychiatry	44	0.52
13	Educational Technology	108	1.29	33	Communication	44	0.52
14	Educational Measurement	104	1.24	34	Multimedia	41	0.49
15	Anatomy	99	1.18	35	Internet	40	0.48
16	General Surgery	89	1.06	36	Problem-Based Learning	40	0.48
17	Education, Medical, Continuing	87	1.04	37	Otolaryngology	38	0.45
18	Pediatrics	81	0.97	38	Resuscitation	36	0.43
19	Videotape Recording	80	0.95	39	Neurosurgery	34	0.41
20	Printing, Three-Dimensional	79	0.94	40	User-Computer Interface	34	0.41

Figure 28　Highest frequent MeSH terms from publications in medical educational technology in the recent ten years（2011–2020）

5. Top 1% most cited papers in medical educational technology in the recent ten years（2011–2020）（Figure 29）

Ranking	Most cited papers	Frequency
1	McGaghie W C, Issenberg S B, Cohen E R, Barsuk J H, Wayne D B. Does simulation-based medical education with deliberate practice yield better results than traditional clinical education? A meta-analytic comparative review of the evidence. Acad Med. 2011 Jun; 86(6): 706-711.	695
2	French S D, Green S E, O'Connor D A, McKenzie J E, Francis J J, Michie S, Buchbinder R, Schattner P, Spike N, Grimshaw J M. Developing theory-informed behaviour change interventions to implement evidence into practice: a systematic approach using the Theoretical Domains Framework. Implement Sci. 2012 Apr 24; 7:38.	523
3	Motola I, Devine L A, Chung H S, Sullivan J E, Issenberg S B. Simulation in healthcare education: a best evidence practical guide. AMEE Guide No. 82. Med Teach. 2013 Oct; 35(10): e1511-e1530.	297
4	Andreatta P, Saxton E, Thompson M, Annich G. Simulation-based mock codes significantly correlate with improved pediatric patient cardiopulmonary arrest survival rates. Pediatr Crit Care Med. 2011 Jan; 12(1): 33-38.	205
5	Hamstra S J, Brydges R, Hatala R, Zendejas B, Cook D A. Reconsidering fidelity in simulation-based training. Acad Med. 2014 Mar; 89(3): 387-392.	185
6	Preece D, Williams S B, Lam R, Weller R. "Let's get physical": advantages of a physical model over 3D computer models and textbooks in learning imaging anatomy. Anat Sci Educ. 2013 Jul-Aug; 6(4): 216-224.	174
7	Jaffar A A. YouTube: An emerging tool in anatomy education. Anat Sci Educ. 2012 May-Jun; 5(3): 158-164.	137
8	Moro C, Štromberga Z, Raikos A, Stirling A. The effectiveness of virtual and augmented reality in health sciences and medical anatomy. Anat Sci Educ. 2017 Nov; 10(6): 549-559.	133
9	Kogan J R, Conforti L, Bernabeo E, Iobst W, Holmboe E. Opening the black box of clinical skills assessment via observation: a conceptual model. Med Educ. 2011 Oct; 45(10): 1048-1060.	127
10	Costello J P, Olivieri L J, Su L, Krieger A, Alfares F, Thabit O, Marshall M B, Yoo S J, Kim P C, Jonas R A, Nath D S. Incorporating three-dimensional printing into a simulation-based congenital heart disease and critical care training curriculum for resident physicians. Congenit Heart Dis. 2015 Mar-Apr; 10(2): 185-190.	107

Ranking	Most cited papers	Frequency
11	Cannon W D, Garrett W E Jr, Hunter R E, Sweeney H J, Eckhoff D G, Nicandri G T, Hutchinson M R, Johnson D D, Bisson L J, Bedi A, Hill J A, Koh J L, Reinig K D. Improving residency training in arthroscopic knee surgery with the use of a virtual-reality simulator. A randomized blinded study. J Bone Joint Surg Am. 2014 Nov 5; 96(21): 1798-1806.	105
12	Khot Z, Quinlan K, Norman G R, Wainman B. The relative effectiveness of computer-based and traditional resources for education in anatomy. Anat Sci Educ. 2013 Jul-Aug; 6(4): 211-215.	98
13	Durning S, Artino A R Jr, Pangaro L, van der Vleuten C P, Schuwirth L. Context and clinical reasoning: understanding the perspective of the expert's voice. Med Educ. 2011 Sep; 45(9): 927-938.	97
14	Hunt E A, Duval-Arnould J M, Nelson-McMillan K L, Bradshaw J H, Diener-West M, Perretta J S, Shilkofski N A. Pediatric resident resuscitation skills improve after "rapid cycle deliberate practice" training. Resuscitation. 2014 Jul; 85(7): 945-951.	97
15	Diesen D L, Erhunmwunsee L, Bennett K M, Ben-David K, Yurcisin B, Ceppa E P, Omotosho P A, Perez A, Pryor A. Effectiveness of laparoscopic computer simulator versus usage of box trainer for endoscopic surgery training of novices. J Surg Educ. 2011 Jul-Aug; 68(4): 282-289.	93
16	Davis C R, Bates A S, Ellis H, Roberts A M. Human anatomy: let the students tell us how to teach. Anat Sci Educ. 2014 Jul-Aug; 7(4): 262-272.	91

Figure 29   Top 1% most cited papers in medical educational technology in the recent ten years
（2011–2020）

6. Highest frequent MeSH terms clustering of publications in medical educational technology in the recent ten years （2011–2020） （Figure 30）

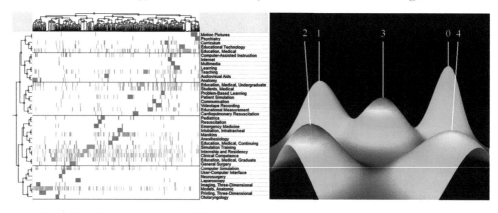

Figure 30   Highest frequent MeSH terms clustering of publications in medical educational
technology in the recent ten years （2011–2020）

Note：The numbers in the right figure indicate the theme categories formed by the Highest frequent MeSH terms
clustering of publications

Through highest frequent MeSH terms clustering，five major themes in medical educational technology emerged：

（1）Application of digital information technology in medical education research and teaching.

（2）Online learning resource construction and teaching impact evaluation for human anatomy.

（3）Application of virtual simulation in medical laboratory education and clinical teaching.

（4）Using standardized patients to develop and evaluate communication skills of medical students.

（5）Application of medical simulation training for clinical practice in graduate medical education.

7. Co-citation clustering of medical educational technology research in the recent ten years（2011-2020）（Figure 31）

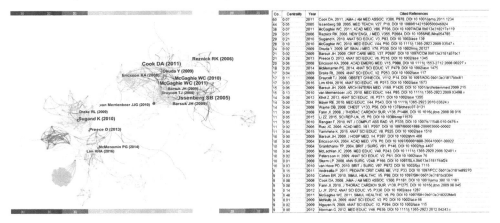

Figure 31　Co-citation clustering of medical educational technology research in the recent ten years（2011–2020）

Based on co-citation clustering, highly cited papers in medical educational technology in the recent ten years were classified into the following seven major themes：

（1）Application of 3D printing, 3D visualizations and other educational technologies in anatomy education.

Recommended reading：

[1] Lim K H, Loo Z Y, Goldie S J, et al. Use of 3D printed models in medical education: A randomized control trial comparing 3D prints versus cadaveric materials for learning external cardiac anatomy. Anat Sci Educ. 2016; 9(3): 213-221.

[2] Yammine K, Violato C. A meta-analysis of the educational effectiveness of three-dimensional visualization technologies in teaching anatomy. Anat Sci Educ. 2015; 8(6): 525-538.

[3] Preece D, Williams S B, Lam R, et al. "Let's get physical": advantages of a physical model over 3D computer models and textbooks in learning imaging anatomy. Anat Sci Educ. 2013; 6(4): 216-224.

[4] Petersson H, Sinkvist D, Wang C, et al. Web-based interactive 3D visualization as a tool for improved anatomy learning. Anat Sci Educ. 2009; 2(2): 61-68.

（2）Development and utilization of anatomy teaching resources based on educational technology.

Recommended reading:

[1] McMenamin P G, Quayle M R, McHenry C R, et al. The production of anatomical teaching resources using three-dimensional (3D) printing technology. Anat Sci Educ. 2014; 7(6): 479-486.

[2] Nguyen N, Wilson T D. A head in virtual reality: development of a dynamic head and neck model. Anat Sci Educ. 2009; 2(6): 294-301.

[3] Khot Z, Quinlan K, Norman G R, et al. The relative effectiveness of computer-based and traditional resources for education in anatomy. Anat Sci Educ. 2013; 6(4): 211-215.

（3）Impact of Internet-based learning on medical education.

Recommended reading:

[1] Ruiz J G, Mintzer M J, Leipzig R M. The impact of E-learning in medical education. Acad Med. 2006; 81(3): 207-212.

[2] Cook D A, Levinson A J, Garside S, et al. Internet-based learning in the health professions: a meta-analysis. JAMA. 2008; 300(10): 1181-1196.

（4）Application of simulation-based education in clinical practice and its impact on health care quality.

Recommended reading:

[1] McGaghie W C, Issenberg S B, Petrusa E R, et al. A critical review of simulation-based medical education research: 2003-2009. Med Educ. 2010; 44(1): 50-63.

[2] Barsuk J H, McGaghie W C, Cohen E R, et al. Simulation-based mastery learning reduces complications during central venous catheter insertion in a medical intensive care unit. Crit Care Med. 2009; 37(10): 2697-2701.

[3] McGaghie W C, Draycott T J, Dunn W F, et al. Evaluating the impact of simulation on translational patient outcomes. Simul Healthc. 2011; 6 Suppl: 42-47.

[4] Grantcharov T P, Kristiansen V B, Bendix J, et al. Randomized clinical trial of virtual reality simulation for laparoscopic skills training. Br J Surg. 2004; 91(2): 146-150.

（5）Research on the relationship between simulation fidelity and learning effect.

Recommended reading:

[1] Norman G, Dore K, Grierson L. The minimal relationship between simulation fidelity and transfer of learning. Med Educ. 2012; 46(7): 636-647.

[2] Issenberg S B, McGaghie W C, Petrusa E R, et al. Features and uses of high-fidelity medical simulations that lead to effective learning: a BEME systematic review. Med Teach. 2005; 27(1): 10-28.

（6）Training and evaluation of clinical skills based on medical simulation.

Recommended reading:

[1] Okuda Y, Bryson E O, DeMaria S Jr, et al. The utility of simulation in medical education: what is the evidence?. Mt Sinai J Med. 2009; 76(4): 330-343.

[2] Cook D A, Hatala R, Brydges R, et al. Technology-enhanced simulation for health professions education: a systematic review and meta-analysis. JAMA. 2011; 306(9): 978-988.

[3] Sturm L P, Windsor J A, Cosman P H, et al. A systematic review of skills transfer after surgical simulation training. Ann Surg. 2008; 248(2): 166-179.

（7）Theoretical research in medical education.

Recommended reading:

[1] van Merriënboer J J, Sweller J. Cognitive load theory in health professional education: design principles and strategies. Med Educ. 2010; 44(1): 85-93.

[2] Mayer R E. Applying the science of learning to medical education. Med Educ. 2010; 44(6): 543-549.

IV. ESI ranking of medical education

ESI（Essential Science Indicators）is a basic analysis and assessment tool launched by Thomson Reuters Corporation, a world-famous academic information database corporation, to measure scientific research performance and track scientific development trends. It is a scientometrics database of more than 12 million articles from more than 12,000 academic journals in the world, collected by Web of Science and including the Science Citation Index（SCI）and Social Science Citation Index（SSCI）databases. From the perspective of citation analysis, ESI categorizes 22 professional disciplines for statistical analysis and ranks by country/region, institution, journal, paper, and author. ESI has become one of the most important evaluation indices used to assess the academic level and influence of universities, academic institutions, and countries/regions around the world.

The total number of citations of an institution is an important indicator of the institution's research ability and influence. One of China's major strategic decisions was to build world-class universities and specializations, which would enhance the overall strength and global competitiveness of China's higher education sector. In this regard, ESI rankings would be an important indicator of world-class universities and specialties. Therefore, we have introduced the concept of ESI ranking into the field of medical education research through cooperation with Clarivate and established ESI statistical analysis and ranking of research institutions for medical education.

By introducing the ESI ranking of medical education research institutions, we can encourage higher-ranked institutions to improve on existing strengths and also find gaps among different institutions, thereby paving the way for future research and practice.

Methods

1. Search Strategy

"Education, Medical" [MeSH] AND (*Academic Medicine / Medical Education / Medical Teacher / BMC Medical Education / Journal of Surgical Education / Advances in Health Sciences Education / Teaching and Learning in Medicine / Medical Education Online / Anatomical Sciences Education / Academic Psychiatry*) [Journal].

2. Time Range:

2011-01-01–2020-12-31.

3. Statistical Method

The total citation count of publications included in the retrieval scope was calculated for each institution. Total citation count reflected academic impact.

Ranking of medical education research institutions by ESI

1. Top 1‰ medical education research institutions by ESI (22/22083) (Figure 32)

Ranking	ESI institution	Country	Number of citations (2011-2020)	Number of publications (2011-2020)	Average number of citations (2011-2020)
1	Univ of Toronto	Canada	15692	1478	10.62
2	Mayo Clin	USA	12293	975	12.61
3	Harvard Univ	USA	11207	894	12.54
4	Univ of Calif San Francisco	USA	10213	1137	8.98
5	Maastricht Univ	Netherlands	7967	717	11.11
6	Univ of Michigan	USA	7868	976	8.06
7	Univ of British Columbia	Canada	7798	659	11.83
8	Northwestern Univ	USA	7409	695	10.66
9	Univ of Penn	USA	7201	862	8.35
10	Univ of Ottawa	Canada	7079	574	12.33
11	Univ of Washington	USA	7066	830	8.51
12	Stanford Univ	USA	6916	778	8.89
13	Johns Hopkins Univ	USA	5830	706	8.26
14	Yale Univ	USA	5617	541	10.38
15	McGill Univ	Canada	5432	532	10.21
16	Massachusetts Gen Hosp	USA	5358	639	8.38
17	McMaster Univ	Canada	5247	555	9.45
18	Duke Univ	USA	5104	574	8.89
19	Brigham & Women's Hosp	USA	5044	556	9.07
20	Vanderbilt Univ	USA	4844	550	8.81
21	Univ of Calgary	Canada	4548	496	9.17
22	Oregon Hlth & Sci Univ	USA	4306	505	8.53

Figure 32 Top 1‰ medical education research institutions by ESI

2. Top 5 medical education research institutions of each continent by ESI Ranking (Figure 33)

Continent	Ranking	ESI Ranking	Part of global top 1%	Institution	Country	Number of citations (2011-2020)	Number of publications (2011-2020)	Average number of citations (2011-2020)
North America	1	1	√	Univ of Toronto	Canada	15692	1478	10.62
	2	2	√	Mayo Clin	USA	12293	975	12.61
	3	3	√	Harvard Univ	USA	11207	894	12.54
	4	4	√	Univ of Calif San Francisco	USA	10213	1137	8.98
	5	6	√	Univ of Michigan	USA	7868	976	8.06
Europe	1	5	√	Maastricht Univ	Netherlands	7966	716	11.13
	2	31	√	Univ of Dundee	UK	3642	200	18.21
	3	40	√	Univ of London Imperial Coll Sci Technol & Med	UK	3205	263	12.19
	4	54	√	Univ of Glasgow	UK	2502	103	24.29
	5	55	√	Univ of Med Ctr Utrecht	Netherlands	2464	203	12.14
Oceania	1	39	√	Univ of Melbourne	Australia	3210	335	9.58
	2	41	√	Univ of Sydney	Australia	3155	367	8.60
	3	43	√	Monash Univ	Australia	2908	390	7.46
	4	73	√	Flinders Univ of S Australia	Australia	1979	196	10.10
	5	75	√	Univ of Queensland	Australia	1960	236	8.31
Asia	1	132	√	King Saud Univ	Saudi Arabia	1073	138	7.78
	2	162	√	Natl Univ of Singapore	Singapore	860	153	5.62
	3	220	√	Univ of Hong Kong	PRC	634	80	7.93
	4	258		Yonsei Univ	Republic of Korea	514	38	13.53
	5	287		Nanyang Technol Univ	Singapore	462	52	8.88
Africa	1	125	√	Univ of Cape Town	South Africa	1111	102	10.89
	2	218	√	Univ of Stellenbosch	South Africa	636	57	11.16
	3	329		Univ of Malawi	Malawi	378	33	11.45
	4	393		Univ of KwaZula-Natal	South Africa	312	61	5.11
	5	432		Univ of Ibadan	Nigeria	288	22	13.09
South America	1	213	√	Univ of Sao Paulo	Brazil	664	137	4.85
	2	357		Pontificia Univ of Catolica Chile	Chile	347	90	3.86
	3	430		Univ of Fed Sao Paulo	Brazil	288	45	6.40
	4	458		Hosp Clin Porto Alegre	Brazil	268	5	53.60
	5	654		Univ of Fed Uberlandia	Brazil	177	12	14.75

Figure 33　Top 5 medical education research institutions of each continent by ESI Ranking

3. Top 20 Chinese medical education research institutions by ESI ranking (Figure 34)

Ranking	ESI Ranking	Part of global top 1%	Institution	Number of citations (2011-2020)	Number of publications (2011-2020)	Average number of citations (2011-2020)
1	220	√	Univ of Hong Kong	634	80	7.93
2	375		Taiwan Univ	326	60	5.43
3	428		Chinese Univ of Hong Kong	289	43	6.72
4	450		Sichuan Univ	273	36	7.58
5	452		Peking Univ	271	58	4.67
6	581		Chang Gung Univ	203	61	3.33
7	676		Natl Yang Ming Univ	171	47	3.64
8	712		I Shou Univ	163	14	11.64
9	867		China Med Univ	130	33	3.94
10	883		Sun Yat-sen Univ	127	35	3.63
11	883		Third Mil Med Univ	127	35	3.63
12	902		Zhejiang Univ	123	15	8.20
13	1008		Capital Med Univ	110	26	4.23
14	1068		Shanghai Jiao Tong Univ	103	31	3.32
15	1134		Fudan Univ	95	42	2.26
16	1242		Central South Univ	86	23	3.74
17	1315		Fourth Mil Med Univ	80	12	6.67
18	1390		Taipei Med Univ	75	38	1.97
19	1505		Hong Kong Polytech Univ	68	11	6.18
20	1563		Chinese Acad Med Sci	65	30	2.17

Figure 34   Top 20 Chinese medical education research institutions by ESI ranking

V. Analysis of medical education journals

Methods

From all journals under the education category (including 41 journals in SCIE and 243 journals in SSCI) of the JCR database, journals on medical education were selected based on the following inclusion criteria.

Inclusion criteria: The journal was considered to be a journal in medical education if 50% or more of its articles published in the recent 10 years (2010-01-01–2019-12-31) were indexed as "Education, Medical" [MeSH].

BICOMB was used to analyze the distribution of high frequent MeSH terms of all journals in medical education in the past five years (2016-01-01–2020-12-31) to reflect research content and special topics of each journal.

Medical education journals（Figure 35）

Ranking	Journal	Database	JCR partition of CAS in 2020* (updated version)	Impact factor (2019)	Country of publication	Number of publications (2011-2020)	Number of papers indexed with "Education, Medical"[MeSH]	Percentage of papers indexed with "Education, Medical"[MeSH]
1	Academic Medicine	SCIE	Partition 1	5.354	USA	4676	2626	56.16
2	Medical Education	SCIE	Partition 1	4.570	UK	2510	1741	69.36
3	Anatomical Sciences Education	SCIE	Partition 2	3.759	USA	680	360	52.94
4	Medical Teacher	SCIE	Partition 2	2.654	UK	3144	1927	61.29
5	Advances in Health Sciences Education	SCIE/ SSCI	Partition 2	2.480	USA	766	388	50.65
6	Journal of Surgical Education	SCIE	Partition 3	2.220	USA	1823	1359	74.55
7	Medical Education Online	SSCI	Partition 3	1.970	UK	514	355	69.07
8	Teaching and Learning in Medicine	SCIE	Partition 3	1.848	USA	569	380	66.78
9	BMC Medical Education	SCIE/ SSCI	Partition 3	1.831	UK	2417	1399	57.88
10	Academic Psychiatry	SSCI	Partition 4	2.148	USA	1563	959	61.36

*SCIE-EDUCATION, SCIENTIFIC DISCIPLINES/SSCI-EDUCATION & EDUCATIONAL RESEARCH

Figure 35　Medical education journals

Highest frequent MeSH terms per medical education journal

1. *Academic Medicine*（Figure 36）

Ranking	MeSH Term	Frequency	Percentage (A)	A/O	Ranking	MeSH Term	Frequency	Percentage (A)	A/O
1	Education, Medical	462	5.27	1.50	16	Attitude of Health Personnel	83	0.95	0.99
2	Students, Medical	438	4.99	1.30	17	Internal Medicine	77	0.88	1.66
3	Internship and Residency	338	3.85	0.55	18	Competency-Based Education	74	0.84	2.52
4	Education, Medical, Undergraduate	269	3.07	1.09	19	Biomedical Research	71	0.81	1.83
5	Curriculum	265	3.02	1.48	20	School Admission Criteria	65	0.74	2.82
6	Clinical Competence	237	2.70	0.75	21	Leadership	62	0.71	2.58
7	Faculty, Medical	200	2.28	2.67	22	Quality Improvement	59	0.67	1.59
8	Schools, Medical	195	2.22	3.05	23	Learning	58	0.66	0.89
9	Education, Medical, Graduate	191	2.18	0.66	24	Licensure, Medical	57	0.65	7.09
10	Physicians	178	2.03	1.61	25	Health Personnel	50	0.57	1.38
11	Educational Measurement	177	2.02	1.58	26	Health Occupations	50	0.57	3.18
12	Physician-Patient Relations	110	1.25	2.60	27	Interprofessional Relations	48	0.55	1.48
13	Academic Medical Centers	102	1.16	5.82	28	Teaching	47	0.54	0.64
14	Delivery of Health Care	94	1.07	0.23	29	Burnout, Professional	45	0.51	1.16
15	Clinical Clerkship	85	0.97	1.96	30	Empathy	45	0.51	1.99

Figure 36　Highest frequent MeSH terms of *Academic Medicine*

Note：A represents the percentage of occurrence of the corresponding MeSH term in all papers published in this journal；O represents the percentage of occurrence of the corresponding MeSH term in all papers indexed as "Education, Medical" [MeSH] in the PubMed database；A/O is the ratio used to measure the publication tendency of the corresponding MeSH term in this journal. The higher the value, the greater the proportion of the corresponding MeSH term in this journal, which then provides reference for medical education researchers in selecting the most suitable journal for article submission.（A/O > 5 have been marked in red, which represent areas of focus, the same below）

2. *Medical Education*（Figure 37）

Ranking	MeSH Term	Frequency	Percentage (A)	A/O	Ranking	MeSH Term	Frequency	Percentage (A)	A/O
1	Education, Medical	233	6.52	1.86	16	Feedback	34	0.95	6.10
2	Students, Medical	231	6.46	1.68	17	Interprofessional Relations	34	0.95	2.56
3	Learning	130	3.64	4.89	18	Schools, Medical	31	0.87	1.19
4	Clinical Competence	129	3.61	1.01	19	Empathy	28	0.78	3.04
5	Internship and Residency	108	3.02	0.43	20	Physician-Patient Relations	26	0.73	1.52
6	Teaching	75	2.10	2.47	21	Simulation Training	26	0.73	0.74
7	Educational Measurement	72	2.01	1.57	22	Workplace	24	0.67	5.39
8	Physicians	66	1.85	1.47	23	Competency-Based Education	23	0.64	1.92
9	Curriculum	65	1.82	0.89	24	Health Personnel	22	0.62	1.50
10	Education, Medical, Undergraduate	65	1.82	0.65	25	Career Choice	22	0.62	0.87
11	Communication	46	1.29	2.66	26	School Admission Criteria	21	0.59	2.25
12	Faculty, Medical	45	1.26	1.48	27	Cooperative Behavior	21	0.59	3.78
13	Problem-Based Learning	41	1.15	2.31	28	Education, Medical, Graduate	21	0.59	0.18
14	Clinical Clerkship	39	1.09	2.20	29	Attitude of Health Personnel	20	0.56	0.58
15	Health Occupations	37	1.03	5.74	30	Medicine	20	0.56	3.82

Figure 37　Highest frequent MeSH terms of *Medical Education*

3. *Anatomical Sciences Education*（Figure 38）

Ranking	MeSH Term	Frequency	Percentage (A)	A/O	Ranking	MeSH Term	Frequency	Percentage (A)	A/O
1	Anatomy	259	17.72	39.13	16	Schools, Medical	16	1.09	0.12
2	Education, Medical, Undergraduate	128	8.76	2.30	17	Tissue and Organ Procurement	16	1.09	24.09
3	Students, Medical	108	7.39	0.10	18	Histology	13	0.89	43.21
4	Teaching	44	3.01	3.54	19	Imaging, Three-Dimensional	13	0.89	14.25
5	Learning	41	2.80	3.76	20	Anatomists	13	0.89	21.26
6	Computer-Assisted Instruction	41	2.80	7.67	21	Neuroanatomy	13	0.89	21.71
7	Dissection	33	2.26	24.58	22	Education, Distance	12	0.82	2.46
8	Curriculum	31	2.12	1.04	23	Social Media	11	0.75	3.88
9	Educational Measurement	31	2.12	1.66	24	Health Occupations	11	0.75	4.18
10	Problem-Based Learning	25	1.71	3.43	25	Academic Performance	10	0.68	5.49
11	Students, Health Occupations	23	1.57	11.14	26	Pneumonia, Viral	9	0.62	0.22
12	Cadaver	19	1.30	21.39	27	Coronavirus Infections	9	0.62	0.22
13	Education, Medical	17	1.16	0.33	28	Anatomy, Regional	9	0.62	8.68
14	Models, Anatomic	17	1.16	7.44	29	Printing, Three-Dimensional	9	0.62	6.58
15	Education, Professional	16	1.09	1.23	30	Pandemics	8	0.55	0.28

Figure 38　Highest frequent MeSH terms of *Anatomical Sciences Education*

4. Medical Teacher（Figure 39）

Ranking	MeSH Term	Frequency	Percentage (A)	A/O	Ranking	MeSH Term	Frequency	Percentage (A)	A/O
1	Students, Medical	396	9.64	2.50	16	Attitude of Health Personnel	46	1.12	1.17
2	Education, Medical	331	8.06	0.02	17	Problem-Based Learning	42	1.02	2.05
3	Education, Medical, Undergraduate	262	6.38	2.27	18	Clinical Clerkship	38	0.93	1.88
					19	Health Occupations	32	0.78	4.35
4	Educational Measurement	150	3.65	2.86	20	Simulation Training	30	0.73	0.74
5	Clinical Competence	146	3.56	0.99	21	Education, Medical, Graduate	30	0.73	0.22
6	Learning	121	2.95	3.96					
7	Curriculum	99	2.41	1.18	22	Empathy	29	0.71	2.77
8	Faculty, Medical	92	2.24	2.63	23	Formative Feedback	26	0.63	3.95
9	Teaching	84	2.05	2.41	24	Physician-Patient Relations	24	0.58	1.21
10	Schools, Medical	79	1.92	2.63					
11	Internship and Residency	69	1.68	0.24	25	School Admission Criteria	24	0.58	2.21
12	Physicians	55	1.34	1.06	26	Models, Educational	22	0.54	2.99
13	Interprofessional Relations	52	1.27	3.42	27	Cooperative Behavior	22	0.54	3.46
					28	Professionalism	22	0.54	2.53
14	Competency-Based Education	46	1.12	0.36	29	Peer Group	22	0.54	2.06
15	Health Personnel	46	1.12	2.72	30	Professional Competence	20	0.49	2.43

Figure 39　Highest frequent MeSH terms of *Medical Teacher*

5. Advances in Health Sciences Education（Figure 40）

Ranking	MeSH Term	Frequency	Percentage (A)	A/O	Ranking	MeSH Term	Frequency	Percentage (A)	A/O
1	Students, Medical	63	5.52	1.43	16	Workplace	15	1.31	10.54
2	Educational Measurement	51	4.47	3.50	17	Faculty, Medical	14	1.23	1.45
3	Education, Medical	46	4.03	1.15	18	Curriculum	14	1.23	0.60
4	Clinical Competence	41	3.59	1.00	19	Clinical Decision-Making	13	1.14	7.44
5	Education, Medical, Undergraduate	41	3.59	1.28	20	Formative Feedback	11	0.96	6.02
					21	Cognition	10	0.88	10.76
6	Schools, Medical	30	2.63	3.61	22	Motivation	9	0.79	6.86
7	School Admission Criteria	27	2.37	9.02	23	Students, Health Occupations	9	0.79	5.61
8	Learning	25	2.19	2.94					
9	Problem-Based Learning	24	2.10	4.21	24	Physician-Patient Relations	9	0.79	1.64
10	Health Occupations	21	1.84	13.06	25	Attitude of Health Personnel	9	0.79	0.83
11	Education, Medical, Graduate	18	1.58	0.48	26	Models, Educational	8	0.70	3.87
12	Health Personnel	16	1.40	3.39	27	Career Choice	8	0.70	0.98
13	Teaching	16	1.40	1.65	28	Patient Care Team	8	0.70	3.85
14	Physicians	16	1.40	1.11	29	Research	8	0.70	5.53
15	Internship and Residency	16	1.40	0.20	30	College Admission Test	8	0.70	15.31

Figure 40　Highest frequent MeSH terms of *Advances in Health Sciences Education*

6. *Journal of Surgical Education*（Figure 41）

Ranking	MeSH Term	Frequency	Percentage (A)	A/O	Ranking	MeSH Term	Frequency	Percentage (A)	A/O
1	General Surgery	388	9.47	8.27	16	Clinical Clerkship	32	0.78	1.57
2	Clinical Competence	371	9.05	2.52	17	Video Recording	31	0.76	5.03
3	Internship and Residency	326	7.96	1.14	18	Personnel Selection	30	0.73	2.75
4	Education, Medical, Graduate	267	6.52	1.98	19	Surgery, Plastic	29	0.71	3.11
					20	Faculty, Medical	28	0.68	0.80
5	Simulation Training	138	3.37	3.41	21	Patient Care Team	27	0.66	2.54
6	Education, Medical, Undergraduate	85	2.07	0.74	22	Quality Improvement	26	0.63	1.50
7	Orthopedics	67	1.63	4.28	23	Orthopedic Procedures	26	0.63	5.31
8	Educational Measurement	65	1.59	1.25	24	Competency-Based Education	25	0.61	1.83
9	Curriculum	60	1.46	0.72	25	Accreditation	25	0.61	2.96
10	Laparoscopy	55	1.34	5.02	26	Robotic Surgical Procedures	24	0.59	3.71
11	Specialties, Surgical	48	1.17	5.87					
12	Students, Medical	42	1.02	0.26	27	Workload	22	0.54	2.59
13	Surgeons	39	0.95	1.77	28	Biomedical Research	22	0.54	1.22
14	Career Choice	39	0.95	1.33	29	Suture Techniques	21	0.51	7.04
15	Surveys and Questionnaires	34	0.83	3.05	30	Communication	20	0.49	1.01

Figure 41　Highest frequent MeSH terms of *Journal of Surgical Education*

7. *Medical Education Online*（Figure 42）

Ranking	MeSH Term	Frequency	Percentage (A)	A/O	Ranking	MeSH Term	Frequency	Percentage (A)	A/O
1	Students, Medical	110	9.23	2.40	16	Learning	13	1.09	1.46
2	Education, Medical, Undergraduate	79	6.63	2.36	17	Education, Distance	13	1.09	3.28
					18	Communication	11	0.92	1.90
3	Education, Medical	66	5.54	1.58	19	School Admission Criteria	11	0.92	3.50
4	Internship and Residency	52	4.36	0.62	20	Stress, Psychological	10	0.84	4.14
5	Educational Measurement	36	3.02	2.37	21	Interprofessional Relations	9	0.76	2.05
6	Clinical Competence	31	2.60	0.72	22	Pediatrics	9	0.76	1.04
7	Schools, Medical	29	2.43	3.33	23	Career Choice	9	0.76	1.06
8	Clinical Clerkship	23	1.93	3.89	24	Attitude of Health Personnel	9	0.76	0.79
9	Faculty, Medical	20	1.68	1.98					
10	Teaching	20	1.68	1.98	25	Biomedical Research	8	0.67	1.51
11	Problem-Based Learning	19	1.59	3.19	26	Social Media	8	0.67	3.47
12	Pneumonia, Viral	16	1.34	0.47	27	Internal Medicine	8	0.67	1.26
13	Curriculum	16	1.34	0.66	28	Physicians	8	0.67	0.53
14	Coronavirus Infections	15	1.26	0.44	29	Staff Development	7	0.59	4.44
15	Education, Medical, Graduate	14	1.17	0.36	30	Computer-Assisted Instruction	7	0.59	1.62

Figure 42　Highest frequent MeSH terms of *Medical Education Online*

8. *Teaching and Learning in Medicine*（Figure 43）

Ranking	MeSH Term	Frequency	Percentage (A)	A/O	Ranking	MeSH Term	Frequency	Percentage (A)	A/O
1	Students, Medical	83	9.79	2.54	16	Preceptorship	9	1.06	14.18
2	Education, Medical, Undergraduate	43	5.07	1.80	17	Problem-Based Learning	9	1.06	2.13
					18	Teaching	9	1.06	1.25
3	Clinical Competence	33	3.89	1.08	19	Pediatrics	8	0.94	1.29
4	Educational Measurement	29	3.42	2.68	20	Empathy	8	0.94	3.67
5	Internship and Residency	27	3.18	0.45	21	Interprofessional Relations	8	0.94	2.53
6	Education, Medical	27	3.18	0.91	22	Career Choice	7	0.83	1.16
7	Curriculum	25	2.95	1.45	23	Attitude of Health Personnel	7	0.83	0.87
8	Education, Medical, Graduate	18	2.12	0.64	24	Quality Improvement	7	0.83	1.97
9	Clinical Clerkship	18	2.12	4.27	25	Health Personnel	6	0.71	1.72
10	Learning	16	1.89	2.54	26	Physicians	6	0.71	0.56
11	Faculty, Medical	15	1.77	2.08	27	Competency-Based Education	6	0.71	2.13
12	Internal Medicine	15	1.77	3.33					
13	Peer Group	13	1.53	8.67	28	Adaptation, Psychological	6	0.71	10.28
14	Schools, Medical	10	1.18	1.62	29	Group Processes	6	0.71	10.16
15	Professionalism	9	1.06	4.97	30	Formative Feedback	6	0.71	4.45

Figure 43　Highest frequent MeSH terms of *Teaching and Learning in Medicine*

9. *BMC Medical Education*（Figure 44）

Ranking	MeSH Term	Frequency	Percentage (A)	A/O	Ranking	MeSH Term	Frequency	Percentage (A)	A/O
1	Students, Medical	609	8.55	2.22	16	Students, Health Occupations	60	0.84	5.96
2	Education, Medical, Undergraduate	371	5.21	1.85	17	Faculty, Medical	59	0.83	0.98
3	Clinical Competence	329	4.62	1.29	18	Computer-Assisted Instruction	58	0.81	2.22
4	Internship and Residency	169	2.37	0.34	19	Health Personnel	56	0.79	1.92
5	Curriculum	156	2.19	1.07	20	Education, Medical, Continuing	53	0.74	0.72
6	Educational Measurement	149	2.09	1.65	21	Professional Competence	50	0.70	3.47
7	Education, Medical	136	1.91	0.54	22	Clinical Clerkship	49	0.69	1.39
8	Attitude of Health Personnel	122	1.71	1.79	23	Communication	48	0.67	1.38
9	Problem-Based Learning	110	1.54	3.09	24	Simulation Training	47	0.66	0.67
10	Schools, Medical	106	1.49	2.04	25	Students, Nursing	47	0.66	5.99
11	Education, Medical, Graduate	103	1.45	0.44	26	Empathy	42	0.59	2.30
12	Teaching	92	1.29	1.52	27	Internal Medicine	41	0.58	1.09
13	Learning	91	1.28	1.72	28	Interprofessional Relations	41	0.58	1.56
14	Physicians	89	1.25	0.99	29	School Admission Criteria	39	0.55	2.09
15	Career Choice	69	0.97	1.36	30	Health Occupations	38	0.53	2.95

Figure 44　Highest frequent MeSH terms of *BMC Medical Education*

10. *Academic Psychiatry* （Figure 45）

Ranking	MeSH Term	Frequency	Percentage (A)	A/O	Ranking	MeSH Term	Frequency	Percentage (A)	A/O
1	Psychiatry	477	13.70	20.04	16	Fellowships and Scholarships	33	0.95	1.67
2	Internship and Residency	281	8.07	1.15	17	Teaching	33	0.95	1.12
3	Students, Medical	151	4.34	1.13	18	Education, Medical, Undergraduate	31	0.89	0.32
4	Curriculum	106	3.05	1.50	19	Career Choice	30	0.86	1.20
5	Clinical Competence	67	1.92	0.53	20	Mental Health Services	27	0.78	12.41
6	Attitude of Health Personnel	57	1.64	1.71	21	Substance-Related Disorders	23	0.66	10.52
7	Physicians	56	1.61	1.28	22	Psychotherapy	23	0.66	12.95
8	Mental Disorders	52	1.49	13.73	23	Depression	22	0.63	6.65
9	Education, Medical, Graduate	52	1.49	0.45	24	Stress, Psychological	21	0.60	2.96
10	Faculty, Medical	50	1.44	1.69	25	Social Stigma	21	0.60	11.89
11	Mental Health	47	1.35	11.48	26	Empathy	21	0.60	2.34
12	Clinical Clerkship	47	1.35	2.72	27	Mentors	20	0.57	2.56
13	Education, Medical	45	1.29	0.37	28	Primary Health Care	20	0.57	1.80
14	Burnout, Professional	43	1.24	2.82	29	Child Psychiatry	19	0.55	13.37
15	Health Knowledge, Attitudes, Practice	34	0.98	2.30	30	Global Health	17	0.49	2.72

Figure 45　Highest frequent MeSH terms of *Academic Psychiatry*

Conclusions

The year 2021 marks the fourth annual release of the *International Medical Education Research Fronts Report*. Through the introduction of ESI， analysis of medical education journals， and introduction of a special series on global research on medical education technology， this new dynamic series of reports holds more authority and distinction. Through literature overview and tracking of research fronts， we can keep up with the pace of medical education development and promote exchanges， cooperation， research and innovation in countries all over the world.